WHAT TO DO WHEN THE DOCTOR SAYS IT'S

Early-Stage Alzheimer's

WHAT TO DO WHEN THE DOCTOR SAYS IT'S

Early-Stage Alzheimer's

All the Medical, Lifestyle, and Alternative
Medicine Information You Need to
Stay Healthy and Prevent Progression

TODD E. FEINBERG, M.D. AND WINNIE YU

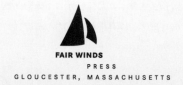

FAIR WINDS
PRESS
GLOUCESTER, MASSACHUSETTS

First published in the USA in 2005 by
Fair Winds Press, a member of
Quayside Publishing Group
33 Commercial Street
Gloucester, MA 01930

09 08 07 06 05   1 2 3 4 5

ISBN 1-59233-161-0

Library of Congress Cataloging-in-Publication Data available

Cover design by Laura Shaw Design
Book design by *tabula rasa* graphic design

Printed and bound in USA

*The information in this book is for educational purposes only.
It is not intended to replace the advice of a physician or medical
practitioner. Please see your health care provider before beginning
any new health program.*

CONTENTS

INTRODUCTION

In 1901, a fifty-one-year old woman named Frau Auguste D. was admitted to a psychiatric hospital in Frankfurt, Germany. She had an unusual cluster of symptoms. While she had no history of prior psychiatric illness, her husband had noticed that Frau D. was becoming increasingly paranoid, hallucinatory, agitated, disoriented, and had increasing difficulties with language functions and memory.

In the hospital, Auguste D. came under the care of Alois Alzheimer, a German neurologist who had a particular interest in the microscopic analysis of brain disorders. He described the clinical features of Auguste D's condition, and upon her death after four years at the hospital, Alzheimer obtained Auguste D's brain for neuropathological examination. In a lecture in 1906, he described the characteristic plaques and tangles in Auguste D's brain that are still considered the central features of the disease that now bears his name.

Nearly seventy years later, when I began medical school in 1974, Alzheimer's disease was considered a rare neurological condition that affected people under the age of 60. If we encountered a patient who had lost cognitive abilities after the age of 65 and certainly after 70, they were considered "senile" and the problem was pretty much accepted as a normal and untreatable part of the aging process.

Needless to say, in the last thirty years that viewpoint has undergone a dramatic revision. We now recognize that except for the age of onset, patients affected early or later in life are all considered to have the same condition now called Senile Dementia/Alzheimer's type. More significantly, we no longer consider the loss of memory and cognition in the elderly normal, or untreatable.

When we established our Neurobehavior Center at Beth Israel Medical Center in New York City in 1986, there were no drugs approved by the U.S. Food and Drug Administration (FDA) for the treatment of Alzheimer's disease. This situation would dramatically change in 1993 when the FDA approved the medication Cognex (Tacrine), the first FDA-approved medication for the treatment of Alzheimer's disease. This was followed by the approval of Aricept (Donepezil) in 1996, Exelon (Rivastigmine) in 2000, and Reminyl (Galantamine) in 2001. These four drugs worked primarily by boosting brain acetylcholine. A fifth medication, Namenda (Memantine), which acts on the NMDA receptor, was approved in 2003. As we shall discuss further on this book, these medications do not cure Alzheimer's Disease, nor are they intended to. However, they have proven efficacy in either ameliorating the symptoms associated with the condition, or slowing down the progression of the disorder.

I'm confident in the ensuing years that additional agents will become available to slow down or even cure Alzheimer's disease. Given the giant steps we have made in recent decades and the extensive research and study that is taking place in laboratories around the world, there is every reason to be optimistic and hopeful.

That said, if you are reading this book, chances are you are afraid, or already know, that you or someone close to you has Alzheimer's disease. This book is intended as a simple guide to help you determine if you do have the condition, and if you do, what you should do about it.

In the first part of this book, we help the reader to understand what Alzheimer's is, the central and characteristic features of the disorder, and how doctors go about making the diagnosis. We next address issues of dealing with the daily challenges of the disorder, namely what sort of lifestyle changes the patient should consider, and how to plan for the future regarding help with self-care and finances. We will also discuss the medications, vitamins, and nutritional supplements that might help slow the progression of the disorder. In this part of the book, we also consider care giver issues that should be of interest to those persons taking part in or managing the care of a person affected with Alzheimer's. Finally, we take a look at the future of Alzheimer's, with a hopeful eye toward a better understanding of the condition and advances in its treatment. Some clinical profiles of patients with Alzheimer's are included that will give the reader a sense of what it's like to have Alzheimer's, and how some patients have learned to cope and adjust to it.

Life with Alzheimer's is not easy, but each year we make progress in making it a little easier. It is our hope that this book will be a first step in that process for you.

—Todd E. Feinberg, M.D.

CHAPTER ONE ❧

What Is Alzheimer's?

Misplaced keys. Forgotten names. The frantic search for a car in a parking lot. In the hustle and bustle of daily life, many of us have experienced these mental lapses at one time or another. We shrug them off and move on, chalking up our forgetfulness to fatigue, stress, or our busy, harried lives.

In some people however, the keys are not only misplaced, but they turn up in strange places like the cookie jar or bathroom drawer. Names of people they know well frequently escape their memories as do names of familiar everyday objects like forks, hairbrushes, and pens. Neighborhoods where they've lived for many years become terrifying labyrinths of confusion. These people may have early stage Alzheimer's,

Alzheimer's is the most common form of dementia in people 65 and older. Dementia refers to any of a number of brain disorders that cause changes in the way your brain functions. To the person experiencing Alzheimer's, the resulting behavioral and cognitive changes can be baffling, even frightening, as the disease slowly robs you of your ability to remember, think, and eventually, perform the functions of daily living. You may experience confusion about the day of the week, or the hour of the day. You may have trouble following simple conversations or directions. Familiar places like your workplace or neighborhood may begin to feel confounding and confusing.

Currently, estimates suggest there are 4.5 to 5 million people who have Alzheimer's in the United States. Approximately three percent of people between ages 65 and 74 have the disease, and nearly half of people over the age of 85 have it. Occasionally, the disease will emerge in adults in their 40s and 50s in a form known as familial Alzheimer's. But Alzheimer's is not an inevitable fact of aging. Alzheimer's is a complicated disease that scientists are working hard to understand.

In recent years, significant increases in life expectancy have lead to a rise in the prevalence of Alzheimer's, which has made Alzheimer's a more pressing issue and a serious health concern. As people continue to live longer, more are expected to be diagnosed with the disease. In fact, if no preventive treatments are developed and the population continues to age at its current rate, researchers estimate that by the year 2050, 13.2 million Americans will have Alzheimer's. That means the numbers of new cases of AD every year will double between 1995 and 2050, according to the National Institute on Aging. In hard numbers, the numbers of new cases will climb from 377,000 in 1995 to 959,000 in the year 2050. By then, nearly 19 million Americans will be over the age of 85.

In recent years, society's understanding of this disease has increased exponentially. Consider the following facts from the National Institutes on Aging's report, "Unraveling the Mystery," which was written in 2002 and published in December 2003:

- Fifteen years earlier, in 1987, no genes had been identified as a cause of AD. Today, researchers have pinpointed the three major genes involved in early-onset AD, the kind that occurs in people under the age of 65. We also have identified a gene involved in the development of late-onset AD, the more common kind that strikes after age 65.

- Ten years ago, the disease could not be reproduced in animal models. Today, scientists have created special kinds of mice that produce the hallmark beta amyloid plaques found in the brains of people with Alzheimer's.
- Only five years ago, the National Institutes of Health did not fund any clinical trials that explored ways to prevent AD. Today, those trials are underway in the quest to prevent this disease.
- As recently as 2001, scientists had no idea how plaques and neurofibrillary tangles, the two hallmarks of the disease, influenced each other. A year later, thanks to animal models of mice, researchers were able to determine that plaques can indeed influence the development of tangles.

And the breakthroughs don't appear to be slowing down. Reports of advances in the study of Alzheimer's have become commonplace on the news and the Internet, and tremendous resources have been allocated to a better understanding of the disease. Just last year, in October 2004, the National Institute on Aging, in conjunction with several other federal agencies, corporations, and non-profit organizations, announced a $60 million five-year partnership to look at neuroimaging techniques and other biological markers to measure the progression of AD and help identify people at the highest risk for AD. The answers would allow researchers to test the effectiveness of new therapies.

Along with all the scientific advances have been several highly publicized battles against Alzheimer's by well-known people like former president Ronald Reagan, writer Iris Murdoch, and actor and activist Charlton Heston. As a society we are slowly chipping away at the stigma of a disease once considered rare and revealing a national health problem that demands full attention, adequate resources, and most of all, compassion and understanding.

If you have just been diagnosed with early stage Alzheimer's, you may be feeling fearful about the future and concerned about how your loved ones will care for you. You may be frightened and frustrated by your inability to do simple tasks. These are all normal reactions to a diagnosis of Alzheimer's.

But being diagnosed in the early stages of Alzheimer's has distinct advantages in this era of greater knowledge. New medications may help slow the progress of the disease, improve your quality of life, and delay the need for nursing home care. It may help you develop behavioral strategies that will help you cope later on as the disease progresses. An early diagnosis also can help you and your family make vital decisions about caregiving, financial and legal matters, and other issues that may become too difficult to deal with later on.

Most important, getting diagnosed in the early stages will give you the time you need to educate yourself about Alzheimer's, to adjust to your condition, and to locate important resources in the community that can help you and your loved ones get through the coming years. The key is developing strategies that will help make the rigors and routines of your daily life a little easier, but also still allow you to live a life that has meaning, purpose, and quality. And perhaps that is the greatest development of all, the understanding that people who have Alzheimer's, especially those in the early stages, are still fully capable of leading meaningful lives and that much can be done to improve their well-being.

WHAT EXACTLY IS ALZHEIMER'S?

Alzheimer's is an irreversible age-related form of dementia that slowly erodes the brain. It robs the person of memory and cognitive skills, and causes changes in personality and behavior. On average, people who have Alzheimer's live eight to ten years after they're diagnosed, though the disease can in some cases linger for up to twenty years.

The disease got its name from a German physician named Alois Alzheimer, who had been treating a woman named Auguste D. in Frankfurt, Germany. In 1906, at the age of 51, Auguste D. died after suffering for years from memory loss, progressive deterioration in her cognitive functions, and bizarre alterations in her personality. While doing an autopsy on her, Alzheimer noticed many unusual lesions and entanglements in her brain. These lesions and entanglements resembled those seen in older people who had been diagnosed with senile dementia. Since this woman had been relatively young, Alzheimer called the condition pre-senile dementia of the Alzheimer type.

In the century since then, scientists have developed a much better understanding of these lesions and entanglements and given them more scientific names, beta amyloid plaques and neurofibrillary tangles. These pathological findings are now recognized as the classic signs of the illness. But where do these come from and why are they there? In order to understand what goes wrong with the brain in Alzheimer's, and why ordinary tasks gradually become monumental challenges, it's important to know how a healthy brain functions and its role in the body's nervous system.

THE BRAIN: A NATURAL WONDER

Everything we do—from making a grocery list to climbing stairs, from creating a work of art to navigating a car—relies on the proper functioning of our brain. This amazing three-pound organ, which rests within our skull, orchestrates our body's autonomic responses, such as breathing, digestion, and the dilation of our pupils, and continuously processes information we receive from our environment. It alerts us to danger, tells us we're hungry, and governs our emotions. It is also the center of all our cognitive processes, allowing us to learn, remember, and to make decisions based on what we have learned.

The brain, along with your spinal cord, is your body's central nervous system. Nerves that extend from the spinal cord to the far reaches of your body, such as toes and fingertips, make up the peripheral nervous system. This vast network of nerves has the enormous task of constantly receiving information from inside and outside the body, then relaying that information up to the brain so it can respond.

This information travels along an enormous network of nerve cells, called neurons. In the absence of disease or injury, these amazing cells are constantly repairing themselves and have the capability to live 100 years or more. What makes the human brain so amazing is the sheer volume of neurons it contains—approximately 100 billion!

Neurons continuously receive and process nerve impulses, which travel along the neuron and are then transmitted across gaps between neurons called synapses. Once in the synapse, the impulse triggers the release of chemical messengers called neurotransmitters, which then bind to receptors on the receiving cell, where the transmission of the impulse is repeated again. The message, or impulse, continues traveling from one neuron to the next throughout the body until it reaches its destination and relays its signal. For instance, if you fall and scrape your knee, the incident immediately sends a pain signal to your brain.

All of this activity happens in less than a split second and without conscious thought. At the end of this process, the brain has the task of interpreting the message and making the decision as to what to do about this new information. What should someone do about an injured knee? A child who receives pain signals to his knee for instance, may cry and run for his mother. A jogger may pause from his run to stretch. An elderly person may decide to take a pain reliever. How a person chooses to respond depends in large part on the memories stored in the brain that tell her how effective her previous responses were.

A CLOSE-UP LOOK AT THE BRAIN

The smooth, well-coordinated yet complex functioning of the brain is truly a marvel of nature. Like a well-organized corporate office, your brain is divided up into different sections, each with its own set of responsibilities and tasks. The brain is comprised of several main parts:

The Cerebrum

The cerebrum is the largest part of the brain and is made up of the right and left hemispheres. The cerebrum contains your gray matter, which gives its outside surface a grayish-brown hue. It is the center of most of your cognitive processes—efforts like thinking, analyzing, organizing, and decision-making in large part take place here.

On the outer layer of the cerebrum is the cerebral cortex. Higher brain functions, like pondering a complicated calculus problem or deciding which is the quickest route to a destination, take place in this part of the brain. It is here that the brain processes the barrage of sensory information it receives, controls our movements, and regulates thoughts and mental activity.

At the center of the two hemispheres is a thick band of nerve cell fibers called the corpus callosum. The corpus callosum links all the billions of neurons between the two hemispheres.

Scientists believe that each hemisphere processes information somewhat differently. The left hemisphere appears to focus in on details, while the right deals with background, or the big picture.

Each hemisphere is made up of four lobes:

- *The frontal lobe.* Located just behind your forehead, the frontal lobe is largely responsible for your personality. It handles problem solving, abstract thinking and skilled movement.
- *The parietal lobe.* Just behind the frontal lobe is the parietal lobe. Here is where the brain receives sensory information, such as taste, smells, and textures. It also helps you determine your location in space using visual and spatial cues and allows you to navigate your surroundings.
- *The temporal lobe.* At the side of your forehead, just behind your temple is the temporal lobe. This lobe is responsible for hearing, some aspects of language comprehension, perception, and essential memory functions.
- *The occipital lobe.* Behind each hemisphere is the occipital lobe, which contains the visual cortex. This lobe handles vision.

The Limbic System

At the center of the cerebral hemispheres is an area known as the limbic system. The limbic system regulates your emotions, instincts, and motivation. It connects your brain stem to the regions of the cerebral cortex. The limbic system houses several other important parts of the brain:

- The hippocampus is a key player in your ability to memorize, store, sort, and retrieve information. Scientists believe that it is here that short-term memories are converted into long-term memories and sent to be stored elsewhere in the brain.

- The hypothalamus acts as the body's internal regulation system, where hormones, food intake, and body temperature are controlled.
- The amygdala houses the body's fight or flight response system and governs powerful emotions such as fear and anger.

The Cerebellum

Like the cerebrum, the cerebellum is made up of two hemispheres. But the cerebellum is considerably smaller, occupying just slightly more than ten percent of the brain. The job of the cerebellum is to coordinate balance and movement. A steady flow of information about your environment helps the cerebellum determine your movements—the dash across the street just before a traffic light changes, stooping to retrieve a dropped object without falling, or turning to greet someone who's just tapped you on the back.

The Brain Stem

At the base of the brain sits the brain stem, which connects the spinal cord to the brain. As the smallest part of the brain, the brain stem controls our body's autonomic processes, such as our heart rate and breathing. Information transmitted between the brain and the spinal cord takes place in the brain stem, too. In addition, the brain stem controls our sleep and dreaming.

The Thalamus

On its way to the cerebral cortex, all sensory information passes through the thalamus. There, information is processed, prioritized and sent elsewhere in the brain.

THE AGING BRAIN

Many parts of your body change as you age. Your bones become more brittle as the production of bone-building osteoclasts slows.

Vision becomes diminished as your eyes weaken. Your skin loses its elasticity and wrinkles more easily.

Over time, your brain changes as well. Nerve cells, unlike other cells of our body, have limited capacities to regenerate. Those that exist may shrink in size. Synapses that allow for proper communication between cells may disappear, and certain neurotransmitters become blocked. The brain shrinks in size. All these changes may diminish your ability to learn new tasks, as your short-term memory becomes less capable of storing information. You may have a harder time paying attention. In addition, you may notice that you are less coordinated, less balanced, and more clumsy.

Though you may be horrified by your inability to recall details or to learn new skills, none of these diminished abilities are life-threatening. In fact, all these changes are normal. What occurs in Alzheimer's disease however, is not a normal part of the aging process.

THE BRAIN WITH ALZHEIMER'S

In people who have Alzheimer's, the neurons become disabled. For starters, Alzheimer's interferes with the neuron's ability to produce the energy they need to do their work, a process known as metabolism. Neurons derive energy from oxygen and glucose—a sugar found in your blood—which is made available through the bloodstream. Without this energy, neurons can no longer communicate with one another and carry impulses to other neurons. They also lose the ability to repair themselves, which ultimately causes them to die.

Exactly what interferes with the functioning of the neurons is unclear, and the rate at which the disease progresses also varies a great deal. But the brains of all people with Alzheimer's do share some common characteristics. Whether these changes in the brain are the cause of Alzheimer's or the result of the disease remains a mystery, but these are two common traits:

Beta Amyloid Plaques

Tucked in the spaces between neurons are thick, sticky deposits of plaque, made up primarily of a substance called beta amyloid. The plaque also contains other proteins, neuron remnants, and immune cells known as microglia, which surround and digest damaged cells or foreign substances that cause inflammation.

Beta amyloid is a protein fragment that has been snipped from a larger protein called aymloid precursor protein (APP), a substance believed to play a role in the growth and survival of neurons. APP rests partly inside a cell and partly outside of it. The part on the outside of the cell is then clipped by any of three different enzymes, substances that speed up or cause a chemical reaction. Most of the resulting segments are soluble, or dissolvable, but some, namely the beta amyloid protein fragments are less soluble and stickier.

As their numbers increase, these fragments cluster together into larger fragments called oligomers. When the oligomers come together, they become even less soluble and form insoluble fibrillar beta-amyloid aggregates. Over time, the fibrillar amyloid congeals into the insoluble plaques that characterize the Alzheimer's brain.

Neurofibrillary Tangles

Another defining characteristic of the Alzheimer's brain is the neurofibrillary tangle. Inside the neurons are proteins known simply as tau, which help give neurons their structure by binding to microtubules in the cell. Like support beams in a building, tau holds up these microtubules, which allows them to perform the essential tasks of guiding nutrients and molecules through the cell.

In a person with Alzheimer's, tau undergoes a chemical change. It breaks down, causing the microtubules to disintegrate and the cell structure to collapse. Rather than bind to microtubules, tau binds to other threads of tau, creating neurofibrillary tangles. At first, it's believed, these tangles may cause poor communication among nerve cells. Later on, they cause the cells to die.

THE CAUSES OF AD

No one knows exactly what triggers the disease process in Alzheimer's, but most experts would agree that genetics play a role. In fact, approximately 30 percent of all people with AD have a family history of dementia. On the other hand, that leaves 70 percent of people who do not have a family history of dementia, which suggests that other factors are at work as well in the development of Alzheimer's.

Genetics

The role of genes is most evident when you consider the family history of people who develop early-onset Alzheimer's, the kind that begins before age 65. People who have early-onset Alzheimer's tend to have a strong family history for the disease.

The strong family connection prompted scientists to look more closely at genetics as a cause of AD. What they discovered was that people who have early-onset AD have mutations—unexpected changes in a single gene or in sections of chromosomes—in one of three genes, while those with late-onset AD were likely to carry a variant of a gene called apolipoprotein E epsilon-4, or APOE-4.

The APP Gene on Chromosome 21

The APP gene is responsible for making APP, the membrane protein that gets lodged between the inside and outside of the cell. The mutations associated with Alzheimer's occur on the part of the APP that's sticking out of the cell, which causes the formation of excess beta-amyloid plaques.

People who have Down syndrome carry an extra copy of chromosome 21, which automatically means they produce more APP. Not surprisingly then, autopsies done on people with Down syndrome have revealed changes in the brain similar to those seen in people with Alzheimer's. People with Down syndrome are also generally younger when they develop AD, with symptoms appearing in their 40s and 50s. Approximately 25 percent of adults with Down syndrome aged 40 and older have Alzheimer's. By age 60, the percentage rises to 65 percent. But oddly enough, not everyone with Down syndrome will develop Alzheimer's.

The Presenilin Genes

The presenilin 1 gene on chromosome 14 and the presenilin 2 gene on chromosome 1 are responsible for the clipping of APP into plaque-producing fragments. There are more than thirty different mutations of these proteins, which can trigger early-onset AD. These mutations promote the production of a specific kind of beta amyloid that is stickier and more prone to producing plaques. The presenilin genes have a strong connection to familial forms of AD, in which the disease strikes several members of the same family. A child whose parent had early-onset Alzheimer's has a 50 percent chance of getting the disease, too.

Apolipoprotein E

Every person has APOE, which helps transport cholesterol in the blood. The APOE gene has three naturally occurring variants, or alleles, epsilon-2, epsilon-3 and epsilon-4. Carrying one or two variants of epsilon-4 increases the chances that you'll develop late-onset AD. Scientists believe that APOE epsilon-4 is less effective at dissolving beta amyloid from the brain than the other alleles.

OTHER POSSIBLE CAUSES

Genetics may influence your predisposition toward getting Alzheimer's and they may even be involved in the development of plaques and neurofibrillary tangles. But at the moment, no one knows exactly what causes the brain to deteriorate in the person with Alzheimer's. Some experts believe that beta-amyloid plaques themselves are the cause of AD, while others point to neurofibrillary tangles as the culprit behind the disease process.

There is also speculation that inflammation may play a role in the development of Alzheimer's. Inflammation is a normal response by the immune system to injuries and foreign invaders such as cuts, viruses, and disease. Studies have found that middle aged adults with higher than normal levels of C-reactive protein, a substance produced during the inflammatory process, were more likely to develop AD later on. But there is disagreement as to whether inflammation is helpful or harmful to the brain and the destructive processes in AD. Some experts believe inflammation is damaging and ultimately causes the death of neurons. Others believe that the inflammation in AD is actually the body's attempt to heal itself by combating the buildup of plaque.

Another possible cause may be oxidative stress. Excess production of beta amyloid and inflammation can damage the mitochondria of cells, triggering the overproduction of highly reactive molecules called free radicals. Normal amounts of free radicals can help the body fend off infection. But too many of them can cause damage to the cell structure, which results in tissue breakdown and DNA damage.

OTHER RISK FACTORS FOR ALZHEIMER'S

Since there is no single cause of Alzheimer's, it's important to understand risk factors other than genetic ones that may increase your odds of developing the disease. We already know that a family history of disease raises the odds that you'll get AD. But just because a family member has AD doesn't mean you'll get it. It only means that your chances are higher than the next person who has no relative with AD. Clearly, other factors are also involved.

Age

No doubt about it, the number one risk factor for AD is advancing age. Experts estimate that for every five-year age group over the age of 65, the percentage of people with Alzheimer's doubles. By the age of 85, your odds of developing Alzheimer's climbs to 50 percent.

It's normal to experience a decline in memory and cognitive function as you get older, but not everyone gets Alzheimer's simply because they age. That's why scientists know there are other factors at work in the disease process.

Head Injury

Experts have known for years that boxers are prone to memory problems caused by years of fighting in the ring. But research is now starting to uncover a link between head trauma and the development of Alzheimer's. A study by researchers at the University of Pennsylvania in 2002 found that mild, repetitive head injuries accelerate the onset of AD by increasing free radical damage and the formation of plaque-like deposits of amyloid proteins. Other studies have found a link between head trauma and Parkinson's disease, another form of dementia. Though scientists have yet to determine how strong the connection is, research strongly suggests that head injuries do raise the risk for developing AD.

Cardiovascular Disease

Most people know that having high cholesterol and high blood pressure puts them at risk for conditions like cardiovascular disease and diabetes. But recent research is showing that these same risk factors may also play a role in causing Alzheimer's. These conditions can damage blood vessels, which supply oxygen to the brain, thereby disrupting important neural circuits that we use to perform cognitive functions. Studies done on mice have shown that animals fed diets rich in fat and cholesterol had more beta amyloid plaques in their brain than those eating standard food. And a study by researchers at Columbia University found that a higher intake of fats and calories over time was associated with a greater risk for AD in people carrying the APOE (epsilon) 4 allele.

Strokes

When the arteries supplying blood to the brain suffers a blockage or a leak, the brain can't get the oxygen and glucose it needs to function properly. This is known as a stroke. Studies suggest that people who have experienced strokes are more likely to develop symptoms of Alzheimer's as well as a condition known as vascular dementia. Since the likelihood of having a stroke is influenced by blood pressure and smoking, there is at least a possibility that some people may be able to prevent Alzheimer's—or minimize its impact—by watching their blood pressure and not smoking, factors that raise the likelihood of a stroke.

Poor Education

Studies on nuns have found some intriguing results that link education with the likelihood of developing Alzheimer's. Researchers involved in the project, which is known as the Nun Study, examined autobiographical essays that the nuns wrote about themselves at the time they entered the convent. On average, the nuns were 22 years old. The essays were measured for density of ideas—the number of ideas per ten words—and grammatical complexity.

The nuns had all agreed to donate their brains to research upon their deaths. When they died the scientists found that nuns who had earlier written essays rich in ideas had fewer neurofibrillary tangles in their brains. Meanwhile, those whose essays were less idea-rich were more likely to have these tangles.

Subsequent studies have suggested that low levels of education as well as lower socioeconomic status might be associated with Alzheimer's. Likewise, people who are better educated and who are at the higher tiers of socioeconomic strata may enjoy some protection from Alzheimer's. Experts believe that somehow the cognitive functioning required of intellectual pursuits may foster more neuronal connections.

However, education obviously cannot protect everyone from AD. Even highly educated people like the writer Iris Murdoch and those with high socioeconomic status like former President Reagan were not able to escape Alzheimer's grasp.

Female Gender

Studies suggest that women are more likely to develop Alzheimer's than men. Though the reasons for this are unclear, it may, at least in part, be due to the fact that women outlive men. According to the Centers for Disease Control, women have a life expectancy of about 80 years, while men have a life expectancy of 74 years.

Clearly, these are not the only risk factors for Alzheimer's. Not everyone who gets AD is poorly educated, female, or elderly. And not everyone has a history of cardiovascular disease, stroke, or head injury. Scientists all around the world are exploring the influence of depression, chemicals, environmental toxins, and cigarette smoking. They're also examining the impact of lifestyle, especially the foods we eat and the exercise—or lack of it—we do. By pinning down specific risk factors that raise your odds for developing AD, there's the hope and prospect that the disease might someday, somehow be preventable.

IN THE MEANTIME

If you've been told you're in the early stages of Alzheimer's or are concerned that you might have Alzheimer's, you've taken an important step toward understanding your condition by reading this book. You've set out to learn more about this baffling disease, to understand what it is, why it's happening to you, and what you can do to take control of the situation. Only by educating yourself are you better able to manage your condition.

So while it's true that Alzheimer's is an irreversible, progressive form of dementia, you may also be surprised to learn that there are factors that can influence the pace at which AD progresses, factors that you can actually control. There are also things you can do to make it easier for you to accept your condition and to live with it more comfortably.

Detecting the disease in its early stage gives you an advantage in many different ways. At this point, you can still actively participate in your choice of medical care and caregiving. You can still make practical decisions about your finances, legal matters, and your living situation. You can still participate in your favorite activities.

No, there is no cure for Alzheimer's at the time, and having AD is certainly not easy. But learning everything you can about the disease will help you understand the options and possibilities that you have available to you, options that twenty years ago didn't even exist. Knowledge of Alzheimer's will also help you live a better life. And that can be most reassuring in the face of an uncertain future.

CHAPTER TWO ✑

What Alzheimer's Looks Like

It isn't easy to distinguish the signs and symptoms of Alzheimer's from the normal forgetfulness we all experience from time to time. You enter a room and can't recall why you went there. You're in the middle of a conversation, and you lose your train of thought. You run into a familiar face, but can't figure out how you know the friendly person who is greeting you by name.

Long before you or anyone around you even suspects Alzheimer's, these memory lapses are treated as a part of the normal aging process. After all, it's true that our memories do falter as we age, and these events can occur even in healthy people in their 30s and 40s.

But over time, the forgetfulness becomes part of a disturbing pattern. You may have frequent trouble remembering something that happened earlier in the day. Events that occurred days ago completely escape your memory. Learning and recalling new information becomes increasingly challenging. As the damage to the brain gradually progresses, these difficulties start to become more troublesome and disruptive.

Establishing whether you have Alzheimer's is a difficult task. There is no single test or biological marker that reveals whether you have the disease. AD also progresses differently from one patient to the next, with differing degrees of severity. And although Alzheimer's is the most common form of dementia, there are also several other forms of dementia that AD may resemble.

To make a diagnosis of Alzheimer's then, doctors must instead rely heavily on what the patient tells him and what family members and close friends reveal. Other tools include a neurological exam, cognitive screening exams, blood tests and brain scans. But it's those reports from the patient and family that a doctor typically hears first, which is why becoming familiar with the signs and symptoms of AD is so critical to establishing whether you have Alzheimer's.

AS AD PROGRESSES

Alzheimer's varies a great deal from one person to the next. No two people will have the same experience with the disease, and no two people will experience the exact same symptoms. In some people, the disease may progress rapidly with extreme severity. In others, it may progress slowly and mildly.

The stages of AD correspond to the underlying nerve cell damage that is taking place in the brain. The destruction typically begins in the parts of the brain associated with learning and memory, then gradually travels to parts that affect thinking, judgment, and behavior. Eventually, the damage affects cells that control and coordinate movement.

Some scientists have broken down the stages of AD into three broad categories—mild, moderate, and severe. Other organizations, such as the Alzheimer's Association, breaks down the disease even further, into seven stages. Keep in mind that these stages are loose guidelines, not strict definitions of what you'll see at each phase of the disease. Some people may display symptoms from a more advanced stage at what seems to be an earlier phase. Others may display symptoms from several disease intervals at once.

The following is what Alzheimer's looks like at the three different stages. Since this book focuses on early Alzheimer's, we'll get into more detail about these early symptoms than we will in the later two stages.

Mild AD: The Earliest Stage

Early on, as the nerve cells first begin to deteriorate, AD may present no signs or symptoms at all. Even the person who has Alzheimer's may not notice anything different at first. But as the destruction worsens, and the person moves into this early stage, changes in behavior may become more apparent. Not every person in the early phases of Alzheimer's will experience these symptoms, but they may include:

Memory Loss

Virtually everyone in the early stages of AD will experience a loss of memory, especially of recent events. That's because the destruction of the disease is believed to strike first in the hippocampus, where our short-term memories are stored and converted into long-term memories.

Everyone has lapses in memory. When they occur in someone older, it's easy to dismiss them as a consequence of advancing age. As a result of these memory problems, it may become more difficult to pay attention, to learn something, and to recall a specific name, phone number, or fact. But given some extra time, most older people eventually retrieve the lost memory.

In people who have Alzheimer's, these short-term memories disappear completely. Appointments go neglected. Events of recent weeks, days, even hours, slip away. Important tasks like paying bills are forgotten. Gradually, these lapses start to interfere with daily functioning, like missing an important doctor's visit or having the phone disconnected because of a forgotten bill. Often, these practical problems become the first indication that something is seriously wrong.

At the same time, the person with early AD can usually still recall things that occurred long ago, which are known as remote memories. Names of a childhood friend or the layout of a grandparent's house may remain vivid because the early stage of AD has not affected the temporal and parietal lobes, where long-term memories are stored.

Difficulty Reasoning

Every day, without a second thought, we go about performing tasks that require us to think logically. In the person with early AD, that thought process, which is sometimes called abstract thinking, becomes increasingly difficult. Without it, it becomes hard to do things that involve multiple steps and that require sound reasoning and judgment. Activities like balancing a checkbook, following a recipe, or reading a manual become very difficult. It may be hard to determine what needs to be done with the numbers, and difficult to comprehend the information that's being read.

Poor Judgment

Judgment refers to the ability to do things according to the information you have. Good judgment also requires sound memory, logic, and the ability to reason. For people with early Alzheimer's, those skills are diminished, and they may make choices and decisions that are faulty, even dangerous. People with Alzheimer's may dress in shorts on a winter day, buy expensive objects they can't afford, or donate large amounts of money to unscrupulous telemarketers.

Language Difficulties

We all occasionally struggle to find just the right word to express a thought. But for the person with early AD, finding the right word or phrase may become almost impossible. The ability to say what he or she means becomes diminished as does the person's vocabulary. Instead, the person with early AD may substitute correct words with others that sound like it. She may also stop talking as much in order to avoid the embarrassment of making mistakes, or she may ask the same questions repeatedly.

Difficulty with communication is called aphasia. Losing the ability to speak and write is called expressive aphasia, while the inability to understand spoken or written words is called receptive aphasia. Often, the person with early AD may cover up these shortcomings by smiling, nodding, and agreeing, making this symptom initially difficult to spot. But over time, family and friends may notice the person's withdrawal and suspect something is wrong.

Confusion About Time and Space

It's normal to occasionally forget what day it is, but a person in the early stage of AD may become frequently confused about what day it is and where they are. She may get lost on her own street and forget how to get back home. She may not remember the day of the week or the month of the year. This type of confusion on a regular basis is often seen in early AD.

Agnosia

Difficulties gauging location may be linked to a condition called agnosia, in which a person has trouble using the information he gets from his senses. Often, the sense affected by Alzheimer's is sight. The person with early AD whose visual information is distorted may lose depth perception, misjudge the appearance of objects, and become disoriented while driving.

Loss of Smell

Many people in the early stages of AD lose their ability to smell. In fact, one study found that elderly people with mild to minimal cognitive impairment who could not identify certain smells were more likely to develop Alzheimer's. More specifically, these people had difficulty detecting the smells of strawberry, smoke, soap, menthol, clove, pineapple, natural gas, lilac, lemon, and leather.

Inability to Concentrate

Our knack for following a conversation or comprehending a newspaper article relies on the ability to concentrate. In people with early AD, concentration skills wane. Reading a passage and making sense of it becomes increasingly difficult, and tracking a conversation may become impossible. Even doing something familiar may become difficult, because a person with AD loses the ability to stay focused.

Loss of Initiative

Most people are energized by doing things they enjoy, whether it's gardening, spending time with loved ones, or taking a walk. A person with Alzheimer's may lose her get-up-and-go energy and become very passive. She may spend hours sitting in front of the television, sleep more than usual, and express a lack of interest in activities.

Extreme Mood Changes

It's normal to feel sad or moody on occasion, but in a person with early Alzheimer's, the mood shifts can be sudden and dramatic, often for no apparent reason.

Change in Personality

The extrovert who becomes a recluse. The proper gentleman who becomes brazenly outspoken. The energetic go-getter who stops

seeing friends. Such dramatic shifts in personality are often a part of early Alzheimer's, as inhibitions give way to a loss of control. Some of these behaviors may become antisocial, offensive, and embarrassing.

In some cases, subtle personality characteristics that a person kept under control prior to the illness go haywire. When that happens, a suspicious person may become blatantly paranoid, or an obsessive person may become a hoarder.

Other Signs of Early AD

AD can affect a person's behavior, cognitive function, and personality in many ways. Below is a list of some other changes you might see in a person with early AD:

- Misplacing things in odd places. The person with early Alzheimer's may put things in strange places like a wallet in the freezer.
- Repeating the same phrase or story, over and over again, with no awareness of the repetition.
- Resistance to making even simple decisions.
- Taking longer to do routine chores and becoming upset if something unexpected occurs.
- May forget to eat, eat only one kind of food, or eat all the time.
- May neglect hygiene and wear the same clothes day after day, while insisting they're clean.
- May become obsessive about checking, searching, or hoarding things of no value.

Moderate Alzheimer's

As the disease progresses and more nerve cells in more parts of the brain are affected, the person with Alzheimer's may develop new behaviors and exhibit more personality changes. It becomes increasingly apparent to family members that something is amiss as the person's thinking become even hazier and judgment diminishes. Here's what may occur:

- Less concern for appearance, manners, and hygiene.
- Trouble sleeping or sleeping for extended periods.
- Confusion over the identity of familiar objects and people, such as thinking your wife is your sister.
- Increasingly poor judgment that poses safety risks, such as wandering, poisoning, and falling.
- Difficulties with organized thoughts or logical explanations make tasks like planning increasingly difficult.
- A tendency to perform restless, repetitive movements, like pacing or trying doorknobs.
- Constantly repeats stories, favorite words, statement or motions.
- May accuse, threaten, curse, or behave inappropriately, even in public.
- May make up stories to fill in gaps in memory.
- May see, hear, smell, or taste things that are not there.
- May accuse loved ones and family members of illicit acts that never occurred.
- May need help with basic hygiene such as using the toilet, remembering to drink, and dressing appropriately.
- May exhibit inappropriate sexual behavior, such as disrobing in public or masturbating in front of others.

Severe AD
In the final stage of AD, the disease has eroded the person's ability to think or reason. The most essential tasks of day-to-day living require assistance, and the person's personality may be entirely

changed. In some cases, the person may be bedridden. A weakened body puts the person at greater risk for other illnesses, which is why many people may die not of Alzheimer's but of infections such as pneumonia. Some common changes at this stage are:

- Complete memory loss. No longer able to recognize self or close family.
- Speech becomes increasingly difficult to understand, or may become mute.
- May refuse to eat, chokes, or forgets to swallow. The person may have trouble chewing and as a result, may lose weight.
- May repetitively cry out, pat or touch everything.
- Loses control of bowel and bladder. The person may experience frequent incontinence.
- Difficulties chewing and swallowing causes weight loss.
- May look uncomfortable or cry out when transferred or touched.
- Walking becomes unsteady, even impossible. May be too weak to stand alone unassisted.
- May have seizures, and experience frequent infections and falls.
- Excessive sleep.
- May groan and grumble unprovoked.
- Needs total assistance for all activities of daily living, including personal care, using the toilet, bathing, dressing, eating, and getting around.

SEPARATING FORGETFULNESS FROM EARLY AD

It isn't easy to distinguish the normal forgetfulness that occurs with aging from the onset of Alzheimer's. As we get older we gradually lose brain cells, and our brain processes slow making it harder for us to recall a certain event, a name, or a telephone number at a moment's notice. But scientists now know that these memories are not entirely lost in healthy people. They simply take more time to retrieve.

In the early stages of Alzheimer's, most people have trouble recalling recent events. So while they can still rattle off all the names of their best friends from high school, they will have difficulty remembering where they went for lunch yesterday, what they ate for breakfast that morning, or who they saw an hour ago. These recent memories are stored in the hippocampus, which is where Alzheimer's typically begins.

What also makes AD hard to detect at first is the person's capacity for hiding any memory deficits. In these early stages, the person can still function normally and behave properly. She may be well aware of shortcomings in her memory and make efforts to hide them, sometimes successfully for several years. Rather than venture into unfamiliar places or do new things for instance, she may stick with surroundings she knows and activities she can do well.

In some cases, it isn't until a person is placed in a stressful or unfamiliar situation that loved ones begin to suspect Alzheimer's. The death of a spouse, a trip to an unfamiliar locale, or moving to a new home can bring out the symptoms of AD when the person becomes distraught by the changes they're experiencing. The changes may be so disturbing that the person will display severe anxiety and fearfulness.

Another challenge in detecting Alzheimer's is the inconsistency of the symptoms. The person's memory may be better on some days than others. He may also demonstrate selective memory, recalling for instance, that he has a doctor's appointment next week, but forgetting a lunch date tomorrow.

So how do you know if your forgetfulness is something more serious than normal? Here are some telltale signs from the American Academy of Family Physicians:

- The frequency of your forgetfulness is increasing.
- You're having trouble remembering how to do things you've done numerous times before, like preparing a favorite recipe or paying bills.
- You have difficulty learning new things.
- You find yourself repeating phrases or stories in the same conversation.
- You have trouble making choices or handling money.
- You cannot keep track of what happens each day.

OTHER CONDITIONS IN EARLY AD

Another factor that makes early AD difficult to detect is the presence of other conditions. Often, AD coexists with other health problems that can mimic or resemble Alzheimer's. Many times, it's easy to dismiss the signs of AD as one of these other health problems or to assume the person has Alzheimer's when it's really one of these other conditions.

Depression

An occasional case of the blues is normal for almost everyone. But some people may feel sad all the time, which is a sign of depression, a serious mental illness that warrants medical attention.

In early AD, depression is very common. In fact, it may even be a risk factor for developing Alzheimer's. According to a seven-year study of Catholic clergy aged 65 and older, those who reported more depressive symptoms were more likely to develop Alzheimer's.

Even if you don't have depression, it's very likely that you will become depressed as the condition progresses, and you become increasingly aware of your diminishing capabilities. You may feel anger, frustration, and helplessness as you struggle to cope with your eroding memory and cognitive abilities. These emotions easily give way to feelings of sadness, and depression may set in.

Because the symptoms of depression are so similar to those for early Alzheimer's, it's often difficult to distinguish one from the other or to determine whether the person has both conditions. In addition, the person with AD who also has depression may have trouble accurately expressing himself and describing his emotional state.

But distinguishing depression from Alzheimer's is important, even if both conditions are present. Treatments for depression can alleviate the sadness, and can even improve the quality of life, even if someone does have both Alzheimer's and depression.

So how do you detect depression in a person with early Alzheimer's? According to the Mayo Clinic, if someone displays one of the first two symptoms on this list, along with at least two others, he or she may be depressed:

- Significantly depressed mood, including sadness, hopelessness, discouragement and tearfulness.
- Reduced pleasure in or response to social contacts and usual activities.
- Social isolation or withdrawal.
- Sleeping too much or too little.
- Agitation or lethargy.
- Irritability.
- Fatigue or loss of energy.
- Feelings of worthlessness or inappropriate guilt.
- Recurrent thoughts of death or suicide.

In people who have Alzheimer's, these symptoms are slightly different than they are in those without AD. In general, the symptoms of depression are less severe in people with AD, and the episodes of depression do not last as long or recur as frequently. There is also less likely to be discussion of suicide or attempts at suicide. The key is to identify depression and to treat it as soon as possible.

Anxiety

As many as 70 percent of people with Alzheimer's also suffer from anxiety, a condition characterized by persistent distress. A certain amount of anxiety is normal, and everyone responds to stressful situations with some distress. You may for instance, have anxiety over an upcoming exam, a marital problem, or landing a new job. But when you become excessively anxious about everyday situations, it is considered a disorder.

In people with early Alzheimer's, anxiety may be related to changes in the brain. It may be a result of the stress you experience from not being able to recall familiar facts or your inability to carry on a meaningful conversation. Not surprisingly then, these changes can cause distress. Anxiety also frequently coexists with depression, and may even resemble depression. Both conditions are characterized by irritability, anger, restlessness, agitation, and insomnia. The good news is, treating anxiety, like depression, can help alleviate these symptoms. Often, the same medications used to treat depression can be used to treat anxiety.

Sleep Disorders

Though sleep disruptions are more common in later stages of the disease, a person with early Alzheimer's may also experience problems with sleeping. Sleep disturbances result from damage to the brain's internal clock, so that the person with AD is sleepy during the day and awake at night. In addition, sleep problems are common in older adults and in people suffering from depression or anxiety. Among the conditions that may affect your sleep are insomnia, which refers to difficulty falling or staying asleep, restless leg syndrome, a condition in which the legs have an overwhelming urge for movement, and sleep apnea, a condition characterized by brief interruptions in a person's breathing while sleeping.

A FINAL NOTE

Like any disease, Alzheimer's reveals itself in various signs and symptoms that you and your loved ones must observe and report. But recognizing these signs and symptoms isn't easy. To the person experiencing Alzheimer's, it may be too shameful to admit these cognitive deficits, especially if you've always prided yourself on your intellect. Or, it may be difficult to find the right words to describe the problem, given the memory loss and loss of language skills.

For loved ones, it may be hard to realize that anything serious is wrong. The signs of disease can be fleeting and inconsistent. For instance, one day your mother may forget she spoke to you an hour earlier. The next day, she may recite to you everything she ate for dinner the night before.

Adding to the confusion is the fact that many people with early Alzheimer's work hard to hide their diminished abilities. They may tell you they don't want to take a trip because they don't enjoy traveling anymore when in fact, they're terrified about leaving familiar surroundings. As a result, it may be years before it becomes apparent that something is actually wrong.

But detecting the signs and symptoms of AD is important for your health. Getting diagnosed while the disease is in its early stages will help you adapt to having Alzheimer's before the disease enters its more challenging stages. It will also give you the time to make critical decisions about your care in the future. Best of all, it can help you develop strategies for slowing the progress of your condition.

CHAPTER THREE ✀

Diagnosing Alzheimer's

You're worried. Memory lapses have become more frequent, and you find yourself frequently confused about the day of the week, your whereabouts, and what you did just hours ago. A family history of Alzheimer's has you wondering whether you have the disease. You call your doctor seeking help.

At the moment, diagnosing Alzheimer's remains an imprecise science. Unlike many diseases which can be diagnosed by a marker in the blood or an X-ray, Alzheimer's cannot be fully confirmed until autopsy, when the disease's telltale plaques and tangles can be seen on the brain.

Instead, doctors rely on a combination of patient history—which includes observations by family members and close friends—and various exams, laboratory tests, and brain scans to determine whether someone has Alzheimer's. Taken together, these tools allow a doctor to diagnose a patient with probable Alzheimer's. The sum total of these diagnostic measures produce remarkable accuracy—90 percent of the time, doctors are right when they diagnose someone with Alzheimer's.

If you're concerned at all about your memory problems or those of a loved one, consider consulting a physician. Getting a proper diagnosis helps rule out other conditions that may mimic or resemble Alzheimer's, conditions that are often treatable and reversible. It will also help you secure a diagnosis of early Alzheimer's, which will give you the time to learn more about the disease, adapt to having it, and plan for the day-to-day care you may need down the road.

MEDICAL EVALUATIONS

The following are some helpful tools and tests that a physician may use to determine whether you have Alzheimer's:

Patient History

Most physicians will begin your evaluation by asking about your health history. To get the most accurate portrayal of your health and well-being, you should go to this appointment with a loved one, spouse, or close friend who can also add insight to your health history and provide information about personality changes that you, the patient, may not be aware of.

In addition to establishing basic information such as your age, your doctor will most likely want to know the following:

- Your symptoms. When did they begin? When did you first notice them? Are they getting worse with time? How are they affecting your day-to-day living?
- Other medical conditions you have.
- Your medical history.
- Your current health status.
- Over-the-counter and prescription medications you are taking as well as vitamins, supplements, and herbal remedies.

- Family history of dementia.
- Family and cultural background.
- Your daily routine. Do you work? Do you visit with friends? What are your hobbies and activities?
- Your mental well-being, which includes assessing for depression.

Physical Examination

The physical exam helps the doctor determine your overall health. The doctor will take your blood pressure, pulse, and temperature, and also measure your height and weight. The physical exam helps the doctor rule out other medical conditions that may be causing cognitive problems such as hypothyroidism and congestive heart failure.

Blood and Urine Tests

As part of the process, your doctor may also ask for a sample of your blood and urine. These important laboratory tests can reveal infections, liver and kidney problems, diabetes, thyroid problems, and anemia. Certain conditions, such as megaloblastic anemia, which is caused by a vitamin B12 or folate deficiency, can be detected in the blood and may resemble dementia. Metabolic imbalances in the thyroid, liver, and kidneys can also cause symptoms of dementia.

Mental Status

Using a simple screening test called the Mini-Mental State Exam, the doctor will gauge your mental abilities, namely memory, language, and organizational skills. The test includes questions regarding your whereabouts and asks you to perform simple tasks. It measures and evaluates your ability to remember, understand, and communicate. A low score alone does not indicate you have Alzheimer's or any other form of dementia, but simply suggests that you might.

Neurological Exam
Neurology refers to the study of the brain and nervous system. To get an idea of how well your brain and nerves are functioning, your doctor will check your reflexes, coordination, and motor skills. These exams may help determine what parts of the brain are affected. They can also help determine whether you may have other neurological disorders. Several conditions may resemble Alzheimer's, and they will be discussed later in this chapter.

Lumbar Puncture
Examining the cerebrospinal fluid that supports the brain can provide information about the presence of other diseases. The procedure, which is commonly called a spinal tap, involves inserting a needle into the fluid in the spinal canal. The fluid is removed and examined for conditions such as normal pressure hydrocephalus and brain tumors, conditions that can cause dementia, but which are both treatable.

Brain Scans
Modern science has made it possible for us to view the brain through different imaging technologies. In people with Alzheimer's, shrinkage in some areas of the brain may be detected through the use of these techniques. There are four scans that are commonly used to determine whether someone has Alzheimer's:

- *CT scan, also called computerized tomography or CAT scan.* Unlike X-rays that shoot two-dimensional images of a body part or organ, a CT scan rotates around the body so that images are gleaned from several angles. A computer then processes the information and produces a cross-section of the tissues.

- *MRI, or magnetic resonance imaging.* Using magnetic fields and radio waves, the MRI picks up small energy signals emitted by the atoms that comprise body tissue, then produces images of organs and structures in the body.
- *PET, or positron emission tomography.* A PET scan helps reveal which parts of the brain are working hardest during particular mental activities. PET is a relatively new technique for detecting Alzheimer's. Radioactive material is injected or inhaled into the body, and a camera follows the path of the substance as it settles into the organs. A computer then produces a three-dimensional view of the organ. In a person who has Alzheimer's, a PET scan typically shows less brain activity than that which occurs in a healthy person.
- *Single photon emission computed tomography (SPECT).* Like the PET scan, SPECT involves injecting a small amount of a radioactive substance into the body. The more blood flow there is in a particular organ, such as the brain, the more the substance is taken up. The radioactive substance emits a special kind of energy called photons, which are then picked up by a rotating camera outside the body. The camera takes pictures of the brain activity, which are converted by computer into cross-sectional images and three-dimensional images.

MAKING THE DIAGNOSIS

A doctor will rely on the results of all these different evaluations to determine whether you have Alzheimer's, another form of dementia, or another condition that may causing your symptoms. If Alzheimer's is the most likely reason for your signs and symptoms, the official diagnosis will be probable Alzheimer's since a diagnosis cannot be confirmed until an autopsy is done. To help doctors make a diagnosis, the National Institute of Neurological and Communicative Disorders and Stroke and the Alzheimer's Association have established certain criteria:

- Dementia confirmed by clinical and neuropsychological examination.
- Problems in at least two areas of mental functioning.
- Progressive worsening of memory and other mental functioning.
- No disturbances of consciousness (blacking out).
- Symptoms beginning between ages 40 and 90.
- No other disorders that might account for the dementia.

In some cases, a doctor may diagnose you with possible Alzheimer's. This diagnosis mean that although the doctor thinks your signs and symptoms are the result of AD, he also thinks there is another disorder affecting your condition and impacting the progression of AD.

MILD COGNITIVE IMPAIRMENT

Everyone becomes a little more forgetful as they age, and the brain does indeed undergo physiological changes. In the parts of the brain important for learning, memory, planning, and complex thinking, the neurons shrink and in some cases, die. The aging brain also has more inflammation and greater damage caused by free radicals, the highly reactive oxygen molecules that can destroy healthy neurons.

In some people, memory losses may be more significant than expected for their age. They may have momentary lapses in concentration and orientation. But other aspects of their cognitive processes remain intact. They can think, reason, and carry on the daily activities of life without any problems. These people may be diagnosed with mild cognitive impairment (MCI).

Studies suggest that people who have MCI are at greater risk for developing Alzheimer's later on. In fact, in some cases, MCI may be a precursor of AD since many of the people who have MCI do go on to develop early Alzheimer's. On the other hand, a good number of people with MCI live for years with the condition and never progress beyond it.

OTHER TYPES OF DEMENTIA

Alzheimer's is by no means the only form of dementia. Dementia refers to a whole category of conditions in which the brain is affected to such an extreme that the person loses basic cognitive skills such as thinking, remembering, and reasoning, and can no longer perform daily activities.

Some forms of dementia are temporary and treatable, but others, like Alzheimer's, are irreversible. In irreversible forms of dementia, the focus is on slowing the progression of the disease and treating the symptoms. Among the untreatable forms of dementia are:

Vascular Dementia

Vascular, or multi-infarct, dementia is the second most common kind of dementia and makes up 20 percent of all cases by itself. Another 15 to 20 percent occurs in combination with Alzheimer's. It typically affects people between 60 and 75 years of age, and is slightly more common in men than women.

The condition results from a series of small strokes or changes in the arteries that supply blood to the brain. These strokes and arterial changes then cause clots in the small blood vessels, which lead to problems in blood flow to the brain, a condition called cerebrovascular disease.

The symptoms of the disease are similar to those in Alzheimer's: loss of intellectual abilities, difficulties with language, confusion, problems with recent memory, wandering, incontinence, and problems following direction. The person may also demonstrate inappropriate emotional behaviors, slurred speech, and difficulties performing daily activities.

The risk for multi-infarct dementia increases with a history of stroke, with each stroke causing a progressive worsening of the symptoms. People who have high blood pressure and high cholesterol are also at greater risk for vascular dementia.

Over time, the condition may improve or stabilize. But it may progressively worsen with each subsequent stroke.

Binswanger's Disease

Binswanger's disease is a rare form of dementia that is sometimes called subcortical dementia. The disease, which is a subtype of vascular dementia, is characterized by cerebrovascular lesions in the deep white-matter of the brain. The condition typically begins in people over the age of 60.

People who develop Binswanger's disease often have high blood pressure, diseases of the large blood vessels in the neck and heart valves, and abnormalities in the blood. Symptoms of the disease include memory loss, cognition, and mood changes. People who have Binswanger's may have urinary incontinence, difficulty walking, clumsiness, lack of facial expression, and difficulties with speech. In some cases, the symptoms may appear for a while, and then disappear.

Dementia with Lewy Bodies

When protein deposits called Lewy bodies become widespread in the brain and destroy brain cells, a person is said to have Lewy body dementia. The disease and the characteristic protein deposits were discovered in 1912 by a German doctor named Dr. Friedrich H. Lewy.

No one knows what causes the brain to produce these Lewy bodies, which are small, round inclusions that can be seen only upon autopsy. Lewy bodies are also present in Parkinson's disease, another degenerative brain disorder that causes stiffness of the limbs, difficulties walking, tremors, and impaired speech. The difference is that in dementia with Lewy bodies, the Lewy bodies occur in both the brainstem and cortical regions of the brain, while in Parkinson's, they afflict primarily the brain stem.

Although most people still believe vascular dementia is the second-leading kind of dementia after Alzheimer's, some experts believe that dementia with Lewy bodies holds that dubious distinction. Various autopsy studies suggest that this type of dementia may account for 15 to 25 percent of all cases of dementia. The disease may also occur in people who have Alzheimer's.

People who have dementia with Lewy bodies experience many of the same symptoms as people who have Alzheimer's—memory loss, difficulties with language, reasoning, and concentration. However, unlike AD, the progression of the disease is much more rapid, and the patient may experience fluctuations in confusion from one hour to the next. The person may also experience visual hallucinations, which may worsen during times of extreme confusion.

Pick's Disease
Pick's disease, also called frontotemporal dementia, is a rare form of dementia that accounts for about five percent of all cases. The disease was named for the Czechoslovakian doctor who first saw the abnormalities in the brain that are associated with the disease, which are called Pick's bodies. These abnormalities, which are tangles of tau protein, cause neurons to swell and produce the symptoms associated with the disease.

Unlike Alzheimer's, Pick's disease affects certain areas of the brain, namely the frontal and temporal lobes, and not the entire brain. The disease usually occurs in people between 40 and 60 years of age, and is slightly more common in women than men. The onset of the disease is commonly described as slow and insidious, as the tissues in the frontal and temporal lobes gradually shrink.

Symptoms of Pick's disease include a lack of coordination, the loss of language abilities, the inability to recognize familiar people, places, and objects, and a loss of inhibition. The person may also exhibit mood and personality changes, including greater anxiety, loss of initiative, indecision, and poor judgment. In addition, the person may lose language skills, become socially withdrawn, and suffer a loss of intellectual abilities.

Huntington's Disease

A person who has Huntington's disease may also develop dementia as part of the disease's progression. Huntington's disease is a degenerative brain disorder that involves the progressive wasting away of neurons in the brain. The condition was first described by an American physician named George Huntington.

Huntington's disease is considered one of the more common genetic disorders. The children of parents with Huntington's have a 50 percent chance of developing the condition as well.

The condition begins between the ages of 30 and 45. Symptoms include the progressive loss of mental functions, increasing lack of coordination, personality changes, and abnormal facial and body movements.

Creutzfeldt-Jakob Disease

Until the mad cow disease epidemic in the 1990s, Creutzfeldt-Jakob disease (CJD) was a rare, mostly unheard of degenerative brain disorder. But when mad cow disease swept through the

United Kingdom and struck even young people, scientists discovered that the cause was a variant of CJD, contracted by eating beef that had been tainted with bovine spongiform encephalopathy (BSE), the medical term for mad cow disease. Since then, there have been several other cases in which people contracted CJD and died after eating tainted beef.

Like classic CJD, the variant form brought on by mad cow disease is caused by misshapen brain proteins called prions, which attack healthy brain tissue. After a long incubation period, the person experiences significant and rapid decline in his mental and physical well-being, including profound personality changes, memory loss, impaired thinking, and lack of balance and coordination. Most people die within a year after the symptoms emerge.

In most cases, CJD develops for no apparent reason. But the disease can be transmitted by tainted medical instruments and contact with infected human tissue. In some cases, the disease appears to be inherited.

TREATABLE DEMENTIA

Sometimes, a person may develop dementia as a result of another condition. By curing or at least partially treating the underlying condition, the signs and symptoms of dementia are often partially or completely reversed. Conditions that may cause reversible dementia include the following:

- *Drug abuse, misuse, or reactions.* In older people, some drugs can produce side effects that mimic dementia, especially if the medication is misused or overused. Common medications that can produce these effects include tranquilizers, sleeping pills, and anti-depressant or anxiety drugs. The symptoms typically disappear after the drug use is discontinued.

- *Normal pressure hydrocephalus (NPH)*. Cerebrospinal fluid is a clear liquid in the central nervous system that acts as a cushion for the brain and CNS. It also circulates nutrients and chemicals to the brain and nervous system and eliminates waste products from the brain. When cerebrospinal fluid accumulates and becomes excessive, a person may develop normal pressure hydrocephalus. The condition—which is also known as "water on the brain"—occurs when the flow of cerebrospinal fluid is blocked. As a result, pressure on the brain builds and can damage the tissues, which can cause loss of brain function and produce symptoms of dementia.

- *Head injury*. Any type of injury to the brain including those that occur during a car accident, an assault, or a severe fall, can cause damage to the brain that produces symptoms of dementia.

- *Subdural hematoma*. Sometimes, in the aftermath of a head injury, a person may develop a subdural hematoma, a collection of blood that occurs between the brain's outer covering and the surface of the brain. The buildup is usually the result of a ruptured blood vessel. In the elderly, this may occur spontaneously or after a minor head trauma. Whether the condition is acute and occurs rapidly or chronic and occurs gradually, it is considered a medical emergency. In addition to causing symptoms of dementia, a subdural hematoma can cause loss of consciousness, headache, lethargy, and seizures.

- *Tumors*. When a brain tumor presses on certain parts of the brain, it can affect that part or cause damage to brain cells. The result may be dementia. By treating the tumor with medicine or surgery, the symptoms of dementia can be reversed.

- *Metabolic disorders.* Conditions that affect the way the body performs metabolic processes, such as liver or pancreas disease, kidney or liver failure, hypoglycemia, or chemical imbalances, can produce symptoms of dementia.
- *Hormonal disorders.* Hormones are chemical messengers that play a major role in regulating our bodily functions, including reproduction, metabolism, and growth. When organs that secrete or regulate hormones become diseased, you may develop a hormone imbalance, which can lead to symptoms of dementia.
- *Poor oxygen flow.* Medically known as hypoxia, the lack of oxygen in the blood can cause dementia. The most common cause of hypoxia is lung disease, which can restrict oxygen intake or interfere with the transfer of oxygen from the lungs to the blood.
- *Nutritional deficiencies.* A shortage of certain nutrients, such as vitamin B12 and folate, can cause dementia.
- *Alcoholism.* Long-time abuse of alcohol can cause a person to develop symptoms of dementia.

GETTING IT RIGHT

It's true that Alzheimer's may be the most well-known and most common form of dementia, but as you can see, it's clearly not the only disease that can cause memory loss, difficulties with language, confusion, and personality changes.

Given that some forms of dementia are at least partially reversible, it's critical that you get the most accurate diagnosis you possibly can. It's also important to get diagnosed as quickly as you can since some conditions respond best early on, and irreversible damage can occur if they're left untreated for long periods of time. It would be a tragedy to learn later on that the form of dementia you or a loved one was experiencing was actually the result of a treatable condition.

On the other hand, if you do have Alzheimer's, it's just as important to get a prompt evaluation and diagnosis. Although there is no cure for Alzheimer's, there are medications that can slow the progression of the disease and lifestyle adjustments you can make that will help you adapt to your diagnosis.

CHAPTER FOUR ❧

Who Will Care for You?

When you were younger and healthier, seeing a doctor once a year for a checkup was probably the most frequent contact you ever had with a healthcare professional, except for the occasional illness. Or maybe it was picking up a prescription from your local pharmacist. But if you think you or a loved one has Alzheimer's, you will be seeing a lot more of the healthcare industry. And as you wrestle with the barrage of emotions that having AD can cause, you may be asking the critical question: Who is going to take care of me?

Finding the right care is important for someone who has Alzheimer's. Whether it's finding a competent neurologist to make the diagnosis or choosing the best person to be your caregiver, the people who care for you can make an enormous difference in how you cope with having Alzheimer's. Caregivers can also affect how your disease progresses. In this chapter, we will take a look at the different people you will need to assist in your care.

YOUR PHYSICIAN

One of the most important people who will participate in your care is your doctor. This may be your longtime family physician, or it may be an expert in Alzheimer's you locate in your community. In some cases, if your family doctor doesn't feel equipped to handle Alzheimer's, he or she may refer you to a specialist.

Doctors in several kinds of medical specialties can treat Alzheimer's—the condition is not the bailiwick of one branch of medicine. Who you choose will depend as much on your personal preference and relationship with that doctor as well your insurance plan and the convenience of the office hours. Each doctor however, should possess some level of expertise in Alzheimer's and feel comfortable treating your condition.

Among the medical specialists who can treat Alzheimer's are:

- *Primary care physicians.* Most of these doctors are specialists in Family or Internal Medicine. These doctors are trained in general medical care and diagnose and treat a wide range of disorders. Although primary care doctors are not necessarily trained in a medical specialty, they should feel comfortable working with healthcare professionals who are.
- *Neurologists.* Doctors trained in neurology must undergo extensive education and training in the study of the brain and nervous system. After graduating from medical school, they must enroll in an accredited neurology residency program. After residency training and obtaining a license to practice medicine, neurologists can become board certified by the American Board of Psychiatry and Neurology by passing an exam. Neurologists who have completed their residency may also enroll in a fellowship program, which can provide training to become further specialized in areas of neurology such as stroke or dementia.

- *Geriatricians.* People older than age 65 may want to consider seeing a geriatrician, a medical doctor trained in the treatment and care of older patients. In general, geriatricians are primary care doctors who are board certified in internal medicine or family practice and have received the certificate of added qualifications in geriatric medicine. At the moment, the number of geriatricians in this country is relatively small. As the numbers of people over the age of 65 continues to grow, the need for geriatricians will increase.

- *Psychiatrists.* These doctors are trained in the prevention, diagnosis and treatment of mental, addictive, and emotional disorders. Some may be further trained in geriatric psychiatry, which includes additional clinical and educational training in the mental and emotional health needs of the elderly, These doctors can help care for and manage the needs of older people confronting illnesses such as Alzheimer's and also assist family members coping with AD.

What to Look for in a Doctor

When your health is at stake, finding a competent doctor with the right credentials and training is critical to your treatment and well-being. You want someone who can accurately diagnose your condition and help you handle any problems that come up. Someone who is on top of the latest developments in the field of Alzheimer's—which is under intensive research these days. The doctor you choose to spearhead your care is a critical player on your medical team. Other things you should consider in making your decision might include:

- *Board certification.* Is your doctor certified in the field in which he's working? Board certification ensures that he has trained rigorously in his medical specialty and passed a rigorous exam that tests his knowledge.

- *Communication style.* Good rapport between the doctor and patient is critical to your healthcare. You want a doctor who can explain complicated medical matters to you in a way that you can understand. The physician should be open to hearing what you have to say and to answering your questions as well. It's also important that you feel comfortable in the doctor's presence, so that you'll be inclined to share even the most intimate health concerns. In addition, it's important that the doctor be able to develop a good rapport with your family and caregiver.
- *Location of the office.* Like it or not, the location of the doctor's office can play a major role in your decision. No one wants to drive a long distance simply for a doctor's visit. So make sure the office is convenient. Is the doctor's office close to your home or workplace? Is it convenient for your caregiver?
- *Insurance.* Another practical consideration is insurance coverage. Does your insurance plan cover your visits to this doctor? Does the doctor accept Medicare?
- *Professional affiliations.* What kinds of alliances does the doctor have with other healthcare professionals in your area? Are there other people in the practice who can assist in your care? Is she plugged in to a network of other medical professionals? Who covers for your doctor in her absence?
- *Hospital affiliation.* Which hospital does your doctor use most frequently? Where would he send you for testing or hospitalizations? Does the hospital have a good reputation? Is it convenient for you and your caregiver?
- *Office atmosphere.* Poor treatment by an unpleasant staff may make you less inclined to make necessary appointments.

Long waits may also deter you. While you don't need everyone to roll out the red carpet, the doctor's staff should treat you with professional courtesy.

When you do settle on a doctor to provide your care, make sure the person is willing to devote the time you need to your treatment. They should also be well versed in the treatment of Alzheimer's and keeping up with the advances in medical journals. In addition, they should feel comfortable referring you to other medical professionals when it's necessary. Ultimately, the physician you choose should be someone that you trust will do his best for you and someone you like.

NURSE OR NURSE PRACTITIONER

While the doctor may handle most of the medical matters, a nurse can provide invaluable support for the day-to-day health concerns. So while it's unlikely that you'll actually choose a nurse, you do want to select a physician whose nursing staff meets your personal needs. The nurse should also be well versed in the care of Alzheimer's patients, communicate well with you and your loved ones, and treat you with courtesy and respect.

PHARMACIST

Getting to know the pharmacist is a good precaution for anyone, but is especially important for someone with a chronic illness such as Alzheimer's. The pharmacist can be on the lookout for dangerous interactions between different drugs and also serve as a source of information about how prescription medications might interact with over-the-counter remedies.

SOCIAL WORKER

Some people who have Alzheimer's may need the services of a social worker. Think of the social worker as a referral source, a person well-versed in the services of a community, who can point you to different family service agencies, counseling services, or support groups. Social workers are also trained to provide counseling themselves and can assist you and your family in making decisions.

GETTING THE HELP YOU NEED

It isn't always easy to find healthcare professionals you like and trust, and sometimes, it may take a while before you find someone who makes you feel comfortable. You can launch your search by asking for referrals, calling the local chapter of the Alzheimer's Association, or contacting an area hospital.

In reality, Alzheimer's is a difficult disease to treat. The condition has no cure, and there are few medications that can slow its progression. Instead, patients and their families can simply hope for the best—that the physician they choose will work hard to improve the quality of their lives now and as the disease progresses.

But as the numbers of people who have AD increases, the numbers of doctors willing to work with these patients is growing, too. Ideally, these doctors will work well with the family members of the person with Alzheimer's and also have the technical competence to help the patient pinpoint any physical problems he might be having. They should also be well versed in what the community has to offer to the patient. In addition, they should be able to work well with the caregivers, and be able to help them identify support groups, adult daycare services, and home health support that the person with AD may need down the road.

THE ALL-IMPORTANT CAREGIVER

Anyone who cares for the needs of another person is a caregiver. The needs may be temporary, as in the case of a minor surgery, or permanently, as in the case of Alzheimer's.

Let's face it: no one sets out to be the caregiver for someone with Alzheimer's. It is a task that falls upon someone—or often, several loved ones—who happens to love a person who has the disease. It is also an enormously difficult task, filled with emotional distress, mental upset, and physical exhaustion. And most Americans are well aware of it: A survey by the Alzheimer's Association released in 2004 found that people are just as afraid of becoming a caregiver for someone with Alzheimer's as they are of developing the disease itself.

Who are these caregivers? According to the National Institute on Aging, the vast majority are family members, with the largest group being spouses, followed in descending numbers by daughters, daughters-in-law, sons, siblings, grandchildren, and others. Most caregivers are also women.

Not surprisingly, people who care for loved ones with Alzheimer's spend more time looking out for that person than those whose family or friends are stricken with other illnesses. Early on, the caregiver may be involved in less taxing duties, such as preparing meals, driving the person with Alzheimer's to doctor's appointments, or making sure he takes his medication. The caregiver may also be involved in making important financial and legal decisions, seeking out medical services, and making important treatment decisions. As the disease progresses, the caregiver may wind up handling more difficult day-to-day tasks such as bathing, dressing, feeding, and dealing with incontinence. At the same time, the patient may become increasingly difficult, hostile, and hard to handle, requiring more and more attention and energy from those around him. The burden on the caregiver—who may often have her own family, job, and household to manage—can become intolerable.

Experts are only now beginning to examine the impact Alzheimer's and other dementias have on the caregiver. Studies have found that not everyone responds to the stress of caregiving in the same way. Those who are male, get few breaks from their responsibilities, and suffer from their own medical problems are most at risk for the physical and emotional stresses of caregiving. That's why this book will devote an entire chapter to the care of the caregiver (see Chapter Eight).

For now, suffice it to say that caregiving can exact a tremendous toll on a loved one, especially as the disease progresses. But research has also shown that being a caregiver to a person with Alzheimer's does have its unique rewards, including a renewed sense of purpose in life, fulfillment of a commitment to a spouse, an opportunity to give back to a parent, renewal of religious faith, and closer ties with people through new relationships or the strengthening of existing relationships.

TAKING CHARGE

Perhaps it's your mother who has been diagnosed with Alzheimer's, and you and your siblings are wrestling with what to do next. Everyone is reluctant to step forward and take charge, but ultimately, someone, or a few people, will have to assume the job as primary caregiver.

In his book, *Alzheimer's Early Stages: First Steps for Family, Friends and Caregivers*, Daniel Kuhn writes about the importance of preserving the patient's dignity—minimizing the affected person's disabilities while maximizing the abilities that remain. The task of caregiver, he says, involves not only caring *for* the person, but caring *about* the person, so that the person with AD maintains his self-esteem.

Of course, becoming a caregiver for someone with Alzheimer's doesn't come with a manual. There are no precise directions to follow. There is no educational training that can prepare you for this job. After all, every patient is unique, and each caregiver is different.

But the goal is to always treat a person with respect, to provide assistance whenever the patient needs it without overstepping your boundaries. "If you are assertive without being domineering, helpful without being overbearing, and kind without being patronizing, then the person with the disease is likely to respond positively to your intentions," Kuhn writes.

WHAT WILL THE CAREGIVER DO?

If you have a loved one who has been diagnosed with Alzheimer's, and you're reading this book to learn more about the condition, you are already beginning to assume a role in caregiving. Taking care of a person with AD is unlike caring for someone with any other illness, and your roles and responsibilities will be many, including the selection of medical professionals to care for the person with Alzheimer's.

Early on, your day-to-day roles may be minimal, possibly even familiar. But have no doubt: As the disease progresses, and the patient's condition worsens, your duties will grow. Eventually, when the responsibilities become too overwhelming, you will face the difficult decision of placing your loved one into an assisted living facility or a nursing home.

While it's virtually impossible to outline what every caregiver should do, there are some general guidelines that caregivers should know. In *The 36-Hour Day*, authors Nancy L. Mace and Peter V. Rabins offer some general suggestions for caregivers of Alzheimer's patients:

- *Be informed.* The more the caregiver knows about Alzheimer's, the better equipped she is to cope with the challenges and demands presented by the patient.
- *Share your concerns with the patient.* When the patient is still in the early stages of the disease, you can discuss your concerns

with him and try to jointly manage problems. It is also an opportunity to share your fears, worries, and grief.

- *Try to solve your most frustrating problems one at a time.* Experts say the day-to-day tasks are often the most difficult and challenging. These might include getting your loved one to take a bath, or getting through the preparation, eating, and cleanup of a meal. Rather than try to solve all the problems at once, focus on one thing you can change to make life easier.

- *Get enough rest.* A tired caregiver is a frustrated caregiver who has little patience and energy for taking care of another person. When you're tired, you are less able to tolerate irritating behaviors. That's why it's important to devise strategies to get breaks from your caregiving responsibilities and to get enough sleep.

- *Use common sense and imagination.* As we mentioned before, the job of caregiver cannot be summarized in a manual or guidebook. Caregiving means learning to adapt to all the changes in your loved one. Ask yourself whether certain tasks are still necessary. Look for new ways to get around a problem. Make allowances for your loved one's new quirks and idiosyncracies, especially if they cause no harm.

- *Maintain a sense of humor.* Holding on to the ability to laugh is critical as you embark on the task of caregiving. Although you may frequently feel angry, sad, or frustrated, there will be moments of laughter. Seize them. And keep in mind that the person who has AD also needs to laugh, too.

- *Try to establish an environment that allows as much freedom as possible but also offers the structure that confused people need.* Now is not the time to start new routines or to rearrange the furniture. The person with AD will want regular, predictable, and simple routines for all his activities, including meals, medication, exercise, and bedtime. He also needs to live in an environment that is familiar, reliable, and simple. So do away with clutter, and keep things as they are as much as you can.

- *Remember to talk to the confused person.* Don't talk about him in front of other people. Instead, make sure to address him in a calm and gentle manner. Let him decide as much as possible, and try to explain what you're doing and why.

- *Have an ID bracelet or necklace made for the person.* Early on, get him in the habit of wearing this identifying tag, which should note that your loved one is "memory impaired," and also include your phone number. Although your loved one may not be wandering or getting lost just yet, there's a good chance that he will someday, and this simple tag will spare you from hours of worry.

- *Keep the impaired person active, but not upset.* Try to involve your loved one in simple, familiar activities that he enjoys. Staying active can help maintain physical well-being and helps boost self-esteem by making him feel involved. At the same time, don't expect your loved one to be able to learn complicated new tasks or skills, which can only frustrate him. Some people may be able to learn new tasks or skills if they are simple and repeated often enough. But too much pressure to acquire new knowledge can be upsetting and frustrating. As the caregiver, it's your job to balance his activities.

A FINAL NOTE

The people who surround you as you confront Alzheimer's will be important to how you cope with the disease. Loving, considerate care from a devoted caregiver can make a big difference for people suffering from AD. And having good healthcare professionals, who are knowledgeable and well versed in Alzheimer's care, can help provide the treatments you need to try and slow the disease. They can also provide the support you and your family need to get through the darkest days.

If you've just been diagnosed with early Alzheimer's and have the wherewithal to have a say in your care, begin laying out your concerns and wishes now. Establish early on how you want your care to progress, who you'd like to care for you, and how you'd like to be treated. If you have a favorite doctor, let your family know about him now. Or if you prefer going to one pharmacy over another, speak up now. Having a say in your care will give you greater confidence and peace of mind.

CHAPTER FIVE ✌

Managing the Challenges of AD

If you or a loved one was just recently diagnosed with Alzheimer's, you are no doubt feeling overwhelmed by the news. You may be struggling with some practical concerns that involve your safety and that of your loved ones. Perhaps you will have to give up driving or turn over the household finances to someone else. Maybe you've already had to stop working. Perhaps you can no longer pursue a beloved hobby such as traveling or cooking.

On top of all these practical considerations, you may be feeling self-conscious, angry, and frustrated because your mind no longer works the way it once did. Or you may be feeling perfectly healthy and strong, which makes it difficult for you to even believe or accept that you have Alzheimer's. Perhaps you may even deny that you have this devastating disease. And when you gaze into the not-so-distant future, you may experience anxiety about losing your independence, and tremendous sadness about giving up your job or hobbies you once enjoyed.

There's no doubt: Having Alzheimer's disease will have a profound impact on you and your family. Tackling some of these challenges early on and outlining your wishes now will help you adapt to your condition more quickly and ease some of the stress caused by the disease. In this chapter, we will look at some of the overwhelming practical decisions and emotional reactions you may be facing. Some topics will also feature a section just for the caregiver, who will play a key role in helping you cope with making these adjustments and dealing with these difficult feelings. While it's virtually impossible to cover all the challenges that AD might cause, we will explore some of the most common difficulties you will confront.

DAY-TO-DAY CONSIDERATIONS

The impact of Alzheimer's varies significantly from one person to the next and can strike at different times for different people. But if you've been diagnosed with the disease, then you probably already have symptoms that are disturbing enough to have warranted medical attention. And that means you are probably also facing some decisions about how to live your life in a way that preserves your safety and well-being as well as your dignity and pride. When you have a disease like Alzheimer's, that can be difficult to do.

WHO NEEDS TO KNOW I HAVE IT?

One of the biggest challenges you'll face after being diagnosed is figuring out who needs to know about your condition.

Some people consider a medical diagnosis of any kind beyond a cold a closely guarded secret. Others may feel comfortable detailing the nitty-gritty details of their health and medical history. How you generally feel about discussing your health with friends and family will be a big factor in whether you decide to disclose that you have Alzheimer's.

In reality, keeping the disease a secret at this stage may not be difficult for you. You may still be able to cover up your bouts of forgetfulness and confusion. You may be able to disguise your difficulties with communication by nodding and smiling. You may also be able to drive, work, and carry on your daily activities without obvious signs of a problem. At this point, you may choose to limit the numbers of people who know to those in your closest circle of family and friends.

But keep in mind that as the condition advances, it will become increasingly difficult for you and your loved ones to mask your problems. Memory lapses will become apparent and your ability to do everyday tasks will slowly diminish. Your silence may also cause close family members to feel isolated because they can't share their despair with others.

For some people at this point, sharing the diagnosis is a welcome relief. Once others know that you have Alzheimer's, they may better understand why you are perpetually late, why you forget lunch dates, and why staying focused on a conversation is becoming increasingly difficult for you. That kind of understanding may relieve you of the stress and anxiety of keeping your condition a secret.

Of course, not everyone may respond to your news in the way you hope. Some friends may be terrified of your diagnosis and may begin to distance themselves from you. Others, on the other hand, may offer emotional support and practical assistance. It's hard to know how people will react to your diagnosis until you actually disclose it.

Whether you choose to keep your diagnosis a secret or divulge it to everyone who knows you is something that you and your loved ones need to discuss, with your wishes carefully considered. But keep in mind that keeping your diagnosis a secret can last only so long. Eventually, your symptoms will become apparent and obvious, even to people who don't know you well. At that point, you may have to disclose your illness.

What the Caregiver Can Do

Ask your loved one how he feels about revealing his diagnosis to specific people at this time. Maybe he doesn't mind if his friends know, but would prefer to keep it a secret from his colleagues at work for now. Or maybe he'd rather that everyone know upfront about his condition.

If he's resistant to disclosure, respect those wishes, especially if he is still able to hold his own in conversations on the job and in the community. But do find out when he thinks it might be appropriate to let others know of his condition.

Ask him too, how he'd like the information to be revealed. Some people might prefer telling friends and family in person, in a one-on-one setting. Others might prefer to do it by phone or email. Still others might ask that you, the caregiver, write a letter. In any case, when you do reveal the condition, do encourage family and friends to offer their support through this very difficult period.

HOW DO I TELL MY CHILDREN AND GRANDCHILDREN?

Your initial instinct may be to hide your condition from the young people in your life. But the truth is, the impact of Alzheimer's is far and wide, and can affect everyone in the family, even the youngest children. Exactly how it will affect the children in your life depends on several factors: whether they are your children or grandchildren; how close you are to them emotionally and physically before the illness; and whether they live in the same house, nearby in the same town, or in a faraway state.

Children who are accustomed to seeing the affected relative may be sad about the changes they witness. They may be confused by that person's bizarre behavior, the constant questions, the loss for words. They may also become worried and fearful about other loved ones getting the same disease. They may also feel guilty, angry, and impatient with the person who has Alzheimer's. Young kids may be resentful of the attention the person needs, while older teens may be mortified by a grandparent's embarrassing behavior. If you're the parent, you may not even realize that your child is feeling these emotions. But your child may display behavioral changes like doing poorly in school, not inviting friends to the house anymore, spending more time away from home, or complaining of vague physical discomforts such as headaches or stomachaches.

The best way to allay these confusing emotions is to have open conversations about the disease with your children. Some suggestions from the Alzheimer's Association include:

- Offer comfort and support.
- Provide opportunities for them to express their feelings.
- Let them know their feelings are normal.
- Educate them about the disease and encourage them to ask questions.
- Respond to any questions as honestly as you can and in terms your child will understand. A discussion of plaques and tangles may be too confusing for a six-year old, but simply explaining how grandma has a disease in her brain might be easier to grasp.

You might also want to prepare your children for what's to come as the disease progresses. Offer your child tips on how to relate to the person with Alzheimer's, like speaking more slowly, providing frequent reminders, and accepting that their loved one can no longer do what they used to do. Remind them that the person with Alzheimer's cannot help the way they are behaving and that they are doing what they do because of very complex changes taking place in the brain. Look for new things that the children can do with their loved ones that are less taxing such as watching a movie, listening to music, reading together, or taking a walk.

A good resource for today's computer-savvy children is the Alzheimer's Association Web site, which features a special section for children. The Web site also offers a list of children's books that might make understanding the disease a little easier.

WHAT CAN I DO TO HELP MY MEMORY?

A telltale sign of Alzheimer's disease is fading memory. Everyday tasks that you once recalled so easily now slip from your mind. As a result, doctor's appointments may easily be forgotten, medications are sometimes neglected, and familiar phone numbers become impossible to recall.

In the early stages of Alzheimer's, you can take steps to help your memory by placing reminders around you. Here are some suggestions from the Alzheimer's Association:

- Post a schedule of what you do every day, such as when to eat, exercise, take your medications, and go to bed. Add anything else that you might do.
- Ask a friend or loved one to call and remind you of important events and details such as taking a medication or making an appointment.
- Carry a notebook that contains important information such as phone numbers, people's names, fleeting thoughts or ideas, appointments, your address, and directions to your home.
- Post important phone numbers in large print next to the phone.
- Have someone help you label and store medications in a pill organizer.

- Mark off days on a calendar to help you keep track of time.
- Label photos with the names of people you see most often.
- Label cupboards and drawers with words or pictures that describe their contents.
- Have someone help you organize closets and drawers to make it easier to find what you need.
- Post reminders to turn off appliances and lock doors.

WHEN DO I HAVE TO STOP DRIVING?

If you're like a lot of people, you've been driving for several decades. To you, the idea of getting behind the wheel of a car was always a symbol of your freedom and independence. But now that you have Alzheimer's, you may have to stop driving.

Some people with Alzheimer's will easily acknowledge that they have become hazards on the road. They might have difficulty navigating through familiar places or have trouble remembering what basic parts of the car are supposed to do. Others may be well aware of their shortcomings, but still be reluctant to give up driving. For them, a life without their car represents a major milestone toward their loss of independence.

The truth is, people who have any form of dementia are serious dangers on the road. While the act of driving is so familiar to most of us that it's almost second nature, driving with dementia is another matter. An impaired brain is less capable of making snap decisions when something unexpected occurs. Think of the small child who suddenly darts into the road, or the car that makes a sudden shift into your lane without warning. Driving also requires that the driver be alert and aware of her surroundings and be able to easily coordinate her eyes, hands, and feet. When a person is suffering from dementia, these abilities may be compromised. To make matters worse, the person with AD may be well aware of these difficulties and feel intense anxiety and stress about them on the road. Such feelings will only compromise their driving further. In any case, the person with Alzheimer's can be a serious hazard on the road, both to himself and to other drivers.

What the Caregiver Can Do

As the caregiver, it's important for you to regularly monitor your loved one's ability to drive. For some people in the throes of early Alzheimer's, driving is still something they can do. But for others, it becomes increasingly difficult and unsafe.

How can you tell? According to the Alzheimer's Association, there are five warning signs that your loved one has become unsafe on the road:

- Forgetting how to locate familiar places.
- Failing to observe traffic signals.
- Making slow or poor decisions.
- Driving at an inappropriate speed.
- Becoming angry and confused while driving.

If you see these behaviors in the person with Alzheimer's, you should suggest that your loved one stop driving. If he's reluctant, you will have to take more assertive measures to get him to stop, which might not be easy. Begin with a frank discussion about his driving abilities. Avoid criticizing his driving, but do gently point out that some of his skills are not what they used to be. You might also start getting him accustomed to not driving by offering to chauffeur him places. After a while, he might come to enjoy, and even prefer, the lesser responsibility that comes with being a passenger.

But if your loved one is still resistant to the notion of not driving, you may have to resort to more surreptitious strategies. The Alzheimer's Association offers the following tips on how to prevent a person with Alzheimer's from driving:

- Ask a doctor to write a "do not drive" prescription. By putting the onus of the request on the doctor, the person with Alzheimer's might be less angry with you.
- Control access to the car keys. Stash them in places where he won't look.
- Disable the car by removing the distributor cap or battery. You can ask a mechanic how to do this.
- Park the car on another block or in a neighbor's driveway.
- Have the person take a driving test.
- Arrange for other transportation.

Getting your loved one to stop driving is critical to his safety and well-being, as well as to the safety of others. So if you sense that his skills have become diminished, take action immediately.

WHAT DO I DO ABOUT MY JOB?

Whether someone with Alzheimer's can still hold a job during the early stages of the disease depends a great deal on the type of job he holds. A job that doesn't demand a lot of concentration, memory, and communication skills may still be doable for a while. But if you have a job that requires a lot of concentration, skill and memory and where the health and safety of others are at risk—bus drivers, pharmacists, and nurses, for example—you might have to stop working pretty quickly.

Anyone who is diagnosed with Alzheimer's has to confront the reality that you may have to stop working before you're ready to retire. Alzheimer's causes changes that can affect many aspects of your work life. You may have difficulties remembering and following directions, trouble concentrating and, and possibly even problems getting safely to and from the office.

To figure out what needs to be done, start by talking to your employer about your diagnosis. Some employers might offer to switch you to a less demanding position, cutting back your hours, or giving you responsibilities that are less taxing. You should also talk things over with your physician and find out how long he thinks you can continue working. Other tips about making job decisions from the Alzheimer's Association include:

- Decide with your employer who else needs to know about your diagnosis. Should you tell co-workers? Clients?
- If you do decide to tell your co-workers, let them know that you may become frustrated with yourself when you can't remember information and that, in turn, may become frustrating to them.
- To help you do your job better, use reminders, memos, and a calendar.
- Look into early-retirement options.
- Research your company's employee benefits to see what may be available to you. People who have Alzheimer's are entitled to the same retirement and disability benefits as a person with any other disabling condition. Remember, Alzheimer's is a disease.
- When you do stop working, find an activity you enjoy to take the place of your job. You might also consider doing volunteer work or taking up a new hobby.

What the Caregiver Can Do
Working is a fundamental part of our lives and central to who we are and how we feel about ourselves. Not being able to do your job can be very upsetting, especially in the face of an illness you can't control.

Help your loved one determine if he can still do his job and whether he really wants to keep working. Retiring prematurely can be distressing to anyone, but may be especially so for someone suffering a dementia like AD. If your loved one does stop working, help him find a hobby, activity, or volunteer work to fill his time and help give his life meaning. If necessary, seek out a social worker or counselor to help him get through this period.

WHAT IF I CAN'T HANDLE MONEY?

The simple acts of balancing your checkbook, paying your bills, and managing your finances can seem like monumental tasks for the person suffering from Alzheimer's. Some people may write the same check over and over again. Others may simply forget to pay the bills. Others may become confused by the math involved in balancing a checkbook. Eventually, the person who has Alzheimer's may become irresponsible with money and give away large sums to unscrupulous organizations. You may also forget when you have spent money, and accuse your loved ones of stealing.

It isn't easy to turn over the management of your finances to someone else, especially if you've always been accustomed to handling the household's money matters. Giving up that task may seem like yet another blow to your diminishing sense of independence. But if you are struggling with managing money, it's best to turn over those responsibilities to someone else, namely your caregiver. The inability to properly manage money can make you vulnerable to significant losses that can lead to devastating economic problems you can't afford.

What the Caregiver Can Do

Once you know your loved one has Alzheimer's, pay close attention to the checkbook and how he handles money matters. Watch for unusually large withdrawals from the bank account or excess check writing. You may consider telling someone at your bank about your loved one's diagnosis, so that person can alert you to any discrepancies or unusual transactions in your account.

Be on the lookout, too, for odd behaviors around money, such as unusually large purchases of the same item, the hoarding of cash somewhere in the house, or the inexplicable disappearance of large sums of money.

As the disease progresses, you'll need to find ways to restrict your relative's access to anything related to his finances, including cash, the checkbook, and other financial papers. You may want to consider giving him a small amount of cash to keep in his pocket or wallet, just for a feeling of security and control—and to avert arguments over money. But limit that amount to money that he can afford to lose, which is typically just a few dollars.

CAN I STILL LIVE ALONE?

In the earliest stages of Alzheimer's, you may still be living alone, and you may not want that to change, even after your diagnosis. Although you will eventually need to make other living arrangements, you can try to take steps to ensure that you live alone for as long as possible. The Alzheimer's Association offers the following suggestions:

- Arrange for someone to help you with housekeeping, meals, transportation, and other daily chores. For information about assistance in your community, contact the local chapter of the Alzheimer's Association or talk to your doctor.
- Make arrangements to have all your checks directly deposited into your bank account.
- Find someone to help you with money matters. A trusted friend or family member can assume the legal authority to handle your finances.
- Plan for home-delivered meals if they are available in your community.
- Leave a set of house keys with a trusted neighbor.

Enlist the help of a trusted family member or friend in making decisions and arrangements about future living arrangements. Making some of these arrangements now, before the disease worsens, can help make it easier for you to accept the changes to come.

What the Caregiver Can Do

Assuming the caregiver does not currently live with the person who has Alzheimer's, it's important for her to be on the lookout for signs that her friend or relative can no longer live alone. Every situation will differ. Some people with Alzheimer's will live alone for several years. Others may need to make different arrangements months after a diagnosis. Here are some indications that someone may no longer be able to live alone:

- The person is anxious, fearful, and wary of being alone.
- The person has started wandering away from home.
- The stove is frequently left on, and food is often found unstored on the counter.
- The person has become neglectful about taking important medications.
- The person is emerging from the house inappropriately dressed.
- You notice odors that suggest the person is suffering from incontinence.
- Basic physical, emotional, and social needs are going unmet. For instance, unpaid utility bills have caused the person to lose telephone and heating services, or the person has become neglectful of personal hygiene.
- The disability has advanced to the point where the person is incapable of handling an emergency, like dialing 911 or remembering her address.

Don't wait until a major crisis occurs to move your loved one into an assisted living arrangement. Do your research now, and make preparations while your loved one can still participate in choosing the type of living arrangement he might prefer. Enlist the input of other family members, healthcare professionals, and social workers in the community.

THE EMOTIONAL TOLL OF ALZHEIMER'S

Being told that you have Alzheimer's can set off a range of emotions in you and your loved ones. You may be outraged that you've been diagnosed with a life-threatening illness, saddened by the loss of a once powerful intellect, or frustrated by your inability to perform as you once could. Or, just as likely, you could feel all three emotions at different times. All of these reactions are very normal responses to a diagnosis of Alzheimer's. How you choose to cope with them however, can make a big difference in how you adapt to your condition.

DENIAL

You do not want to admit that you have a chronic disease, so you tell yourself that everything is okay. You feel fine. You can still handle money, drive the car, and go to the store. You can still carry on a conversation with your friends and do your job fairly effectively. But deep down, you know it's becoming more difficult to perform these everyday tasks. In short, you may be in denial.

This simple strategy has enabled many of us to get through some of life's most difficult circumstances. For instance, we might deny that we're unhappily married in order to avoid the economic hardships that can come with a painful divorce. But in some people who have early Alzheimer's, what may appear to be denial to outsiders may in reality be a lack of awareness of the illness. You may simply be oblivious to your diminished faculties and compensating in ways that you don't find bothersome.

According to Daniel Kuhn, author of *Alzheimer's Early Stages*, personal awareness of Alzheimer's fluctuates in the early phases of AD, but is generally lower than might be expected because of the effects of the disease. "Most people don't dwell on their impairments or they find ways to excuse them," he writes. Instead, they begin to gradually adapt to their condition by accepting their limitations and lowering their expectations. But to the outside world, these people may appear to be in denial of their illness.

It's easy to understand why someone would want to deny that they have Alzheimer's. And in many cases, it's okay to be in some denial as you gradually come to terms with your condition. But if your denial is jeopardizing your health and safety, then you may need to talk to a social worker, your physician or a close family member or friend. The sooner you come to terms with your diagnosis, the sooner you'll learn to live with it.

ANGER

Perhaps you are outraged to discover you have Alzheimer's, especially if you've been vigilant about your health. You may feel that life is unfair, and that you've already had your share of trauma. You may be outraged at the fact you can no longer balance your checkbook, drive to the mall, or follow a simple recipe.

Anger over something you can't control is a normal emotion, one you're likely to experience at least on occasion when you have Alzheimer's. The constant presence of an incurable disease can make anyone angry and bitter. As a result you may become easily irritated, even with loved ones who are trying to care for you.

If you find yourself frequently angry, try to pinpoint the source of your anger. Maybe it's the feelings of helplessness. Or maybe you hate the way you can no longer participate in conversations with ease. Perhaps you don't like feeling different from other people. Talk to your caregiver, a social worker, or a friend about your feelings. If you can, keep a log to vent your anger. Consider joining a support group with other people who have Alzheimer's. You will certainly discover that there are plenty of others who share your anger about having this disease.

What the Caregiver Can Do

Whether your loved one shares your feelings with you or not, you will know that he is angry if he is irritable, sullen, and withdrawn. These are emotional cues that suggest inward anger, even if the patient is not outwardly ranting.

To help ease his anger, let him voice his displeasure without any comments from you. Don't give him difficult tasks that may cause confusion, which will only upset the person. At the same time, don't insult him by giving him tasks that are so overly simple they seem condescending.

Also, speak slowly and clearly, and never talk about the patient in his presence as if he's not there. Don't barrage him with too many questions at a time, which can be overwhelming. Avoid startling the person. Offer help subtly when he appears to need it, but don't automatically assume a lack of competence. If the person erupts in a tirade, invite him out for a walk that might help him cool down.

Frequent episodes of anger may actually be a symptom of depression. So be on the lookout for other signs of depression, such as withdrawing, crying, persistent sadness, and feelings of worthlessness. Depression can be treated, which may alleviate some of the anger and hostility.

DEPRESSION

It's not uncommon for most people to feel inexplicably sad at varying times in their lives. But depression is a serious mental illness that can impair the way you function. As much as 9.5 percent of the population or nearly 19 million people suffer from a depressive illness every year. Depression is considerably more common among the elderly and affects approximately 20 percent of people over the age of 55. Left untreated, the condition can have devastating consequences and destroy a person's career, family life, and other relationships, and cause enormous pain and suffering.

In the elderly who have Alzheimer's, depression is even more prevalent, especially among people in the early stages of the disease who are aware of their condition. These people may be feeling depressed because of their diminished capacities for remembering, thinking, and participating fully in life. They may be saddened by their growing dependence on others and their loss of freedom. They may feel intense loneliness from having Alzheimer's and feel isolated from others who are not sick. At the same time, their brains are undergoing some of the same chemical changes that can cause depression, namely a reduction in serotonin, a neurotransmitter in the brain responsible for mood that is associated with feelings of happiness. But not everyone who has Alzheimer's develops a concurrent case of depression.

It isn't always easy to determine whether you're experiencing a short-lived bout of sadness or a serious case of depression. After all, most people suffer from an occasional case of the blues, and learning you have Alzheimer's is certainly enough to make even the most jovial person feel sad. According to the National Institute of Mental Health, there are some telltale signs of serious depression:

- Persistent, sad, anxious or empty mood.
- Feelings of hopelessness and pessimism.
- Feelings of guilt, worthlessness, and helplessness.
- Loss of interest or pleasure in hobbies and activities you once enjoyed, including sex.

- Decreased energy, fatigue, and feeling slowed down.
- Difficulty concentrating, remembering, or making decisions.
- Insomnia, early awakening, or oversleeping.
- Appetite changes or fluctuations in weight.
- Thoughts of death or suicide, or suicide attempts.
- Restlessness or irritability.

If you have five or more of these symptoms every day for at least two weeks, and they begin to interfere with your daily living, you should be evaluated for depression.

Treating depression in people who have Alzheimer's can help alleviate the symptoms. In the early stages of the disease, you may want to participate in psychotherapy. You may also consider talking to your doctor about taking anti-depressants, such as a selective serotonin reuptake inhibitor (SSRI), a class of medications that have been found to reduce depressive symptoms in patients with Alzheimer's. These medications work by blocking the removal of serotonin, in the synapses, or gaps between the nerves. Inadequate amounts of serotonin, as well as other neurotransmitters such as dopamine and norepinephrine are often the cause of depression. In recent years, these drugs have become enormously popular as the medication of choice for treating depression. In addition, you might consider discussing your feelings with a trusted friend or loved one, such as your caregiver.

What the Caregiver Can Do

If you sense that your loved one is suffering from depression, encourage her to talk to you about it. Simply by listening and acknowledging her feelings, you can help her cope with her sadness. You might also encourage her to talk to her physician, a social worker, a clergy person, or a mental health professional who might be able to help her work through her difficult feelings. But as the disease progresses, avoid any formal therapy or group therapy, since this kind of treatment requires the person to remember and process information.

Be careful not to give false encouragement, like suggesting she "get over it," or "snap out of it," or trying too hard to cheer her up. Such statements may diminish the severity of her depression and only compound her feelings of frustration of not being able to get over her sadness.

To help brighten the mood, try engaging your loved one in her favorite activities. Playing music, doing simple arts and crafts, or watching a favorite video can provide a lift for sinking spirits. Minimize her despair by avoiding tasks or activities that are less familiar or giving her things to do that require a lot of concentration. Tasks that have become overwhelming will only serve as reminders of her dwindling capacities.

Help your loved one remain socially engaged, too. Being among friends can sometimes help lessen the depression and distract your loved one from his sadness. But avoid subjecting him to large gatherings, which may be too overwhelming and tiring. Instead, invite only one or two close friends to come over for some quiet conversation.

Finally, if you think your loved one needs medical attention for her depression, don't hesitate to seek out her doctor for help. There are numerous anti-depressant medications today that can make a big difference in her mood. Just because someone has Alzheimer's doesn't mean she needs to live with depression as well.

FRUSTRATION

It's hard to imagine anything more frustrating than not being able to think and perform at the level you're accustomed to operating at. Compounding those feelings of frustration is the inability to come and go as you please and an increasing reliance on others, even for simple tasks like making a purchase, writing a check, or preparing a simple meal.

When you're unable to resolve problems or do all that you once could do, it's easy to become frustrated, annoyed, and disgusted with yourself. You may feel self-conscious and on guard, constantly fretting about silly mistakes and lapses in memory. Such feelings of frustration are common and understandable among people suffering from Alzheimer's. It often isn't until the person with Alzheimer's comes to terms with his limitations that some of these frustrations abate. In some cases, the frustrations may never go away.

What the Caregiver Can Do

Caregivers can play a pivotal role in alleviating the frustration of a loved one with Alzheimer's. For starters, you can try to let your loved one do as much as he can with as little assistance from you as possible. By giving your loved one some control over what he can do and not just focusing on what he can't, you'll boost his self-confidence and relieve some of his feelings of frustration.

Resist the urge to criticize the way your loved one does things and whether he's doing them the way you think he should. As long as your loved one isn't putting himself or anyone else in danger, there's no reason to point out minor mistakes or less efficient ways of doing something. Setting standards above what he can do will only exacerbate his frustration.

Always give your loved one enough time to do what he needs to get done. Whether it's choosing his wardrobe for the day, drinking a cup of coffee, or preparing for a bath, make sure he has ample time to do it, so you're not rushing him and annoying him unnecessarily.

Restrict your loved one's level of activity when he's fatigued. Giving him too much to do when his energy levels are low will only serve to aggravate and annoy him. Try to recognize when he's too tired, and urge him to attempt the activity when he feels more rested.

Creating the right environment can also help reduce frustration. Limit the amount of noise and activity in your loved one's immediate surroundings. Avoid making radical changes in his living space as well as his routine. Try to stick to a consistent schedule, so he comes to know what to expect throughout his day. By making his days predictable and his environment constant, you'll provide your loved one with the comforting routine and consistency he craves.

ALIENATION

People who have Alzheimer's often speak of the incredible loneliness they feel. No one knows exactly what goes on inside the mind of a person with AD, and no two patients are exactly alike. The reaction to having Alzheimer's also differs a great deal from one person to the next. As a result, people with Alzheimer's often feel intensely isolated by their condition, unable to share their feelings with anyone else.

The best way to avoid these feelings of isolation is to tap into a support group, preferably one made up entirely of people in the early stages of the disease. Reading books, articles, journals, and Web sites written by others who have Alzheimer's can also help assuage your feelings of loneliness. Knowing that there are others out there sharing your predicament can provide enormous comfort.

What the Caregiver Can Do

People who become caregivers often suffer the same intense loneliness that their loved ones do, especially later on, as the disease progresses. The good news is, as the disease has become more openly discussed, people are now more willing to turn to each other for support, advice, and comfort. Numerous organizations today offer support groups for caregivers and their loved ones.

Join one now, even if you think you don't currently need the outside support of strangers. Contact organizations like the Alzheimer's Association, the Alzheimer's Disease Education and Referral Center, and organizations that cater to the elderly and find out about local resources. Don't wait until you reach a breaking point or are in such despair that you're too overwhelmed to meet new people. You'll be relieved to find that there are other people just like you and your loved one dealing with the struggles of Alzheimer's.

CHAPTER SIX ⨾

Staying Healthy: Why Good Habits Count

Exercise. Eat your vegetables. Get your rest. We've heard these health mantras all our lives, from parents, teachers, doctors, and even the media. There's a reason why these messages persist— they speak the truth and are critical to helping us sustain healthy bodies and minds.

Now that you have Alzheimer's, you may be too depressed, too lethargic, or too lackadaisical to care about your health. You may wonder why you should bother if your mind is slowly deteriorating anyway. Or you may lack the appetite or the energy to eat well and exercise. But in reality, taking care of your health now may be more important than ever as you begin your journey with Alzheimer's.

Taking care of your overall health by eating well, doing regular exercise, getting your rest, and staying active will give you the physical and mental advantage you'll need to cope with Alzheimer's. Many of these simple stay-healthy strategies can lessen the symptoms of Alzheimer's and prevent complications from other health problems. They can also help minimize your stress and frustration.

Current research suggests that some of these strategies may even help lower the risk for developing Alzheimer's and keep the brain healthy in people who do not have Alzheimer's. One study on beagles published in 2005 found that aging beagles were better able to learn new tricks if they ate plenty of fruits and vegetables, got regular exercise, and played with other dogs and interesting toys. Dogs that followed all three healthy strategies did better at learning difficult tasks than the dogs who received standard care. While dogs are certainly not people, they do experience the same age-related cognitive declines that people do, which suggests that these results may be relevant to us.

EATING FOR THE BRAIN

For many of us, few things are more pleasurable than devouring our favorite foods, be it a hot fudge sundae, a delectable Thanksgiving dinner, or a steamy bowl of noodle soup. Eating is one of life's greatest sources of pleasure. It also provides our bodies with essential energy and powers our ability to move, think, and do all that we do.

Research in recent years has found that our diets have a profound impact on our brains. In reality, the word on healthy eating for the brain is nothing new. Many of the messages that we hear about preventing diabetes, staying slim, and avoiding cardiovascular disease are the same ones that apply to eating well for the brain. But these messages are always well worth repeating.

Go for the Color

Fruits and vegetables that are resplendent in their hues should be the part of any brain-healthy diet. These foods are rich in anti-oxidants that can prevent oxidative damage to brain cells caused by disease-promoting free radicals. Vegetables dense in anti-oxidants include kale, spinach, broccoli, brussel sprouts, red peppers, corn, eggplant, and onions. Fruits that have a lot of antioxidants include blueberries, strawberries, plums, blackberries, oranges, red grapes, cherries, raspberries, cranberries, and prunes.

Make Fish a Part of Your Diet

Certain fish, such as halibut, mackerel, salmon, and tuna, are rich in omega-3 fatty acids, healthy fats with anti-inflammatory effects that not only lower the risk for cardiovascular disease but may keep Alzheimer's at bay. A study by the Rush Institute for Healthy Aging looked at the fish-eating habits of elderly people between ages 65 and 94 and found that those who ate at least one fish meal a week were less likely to develop Alzheimer's.

But choose your fish carefully. Some fish, especially larger ones like swordfish and tuna, are higher in mercury content than others. Others, including canned light tuna, shrimp, and salmon, are lower in mercury. Although mercury poses the greatest risk to young children, pregnant women, and women in their childbearing years, everyone should still limit their intake of these kinds of fish. For more information about fish and mercury, check out the Environmental Protection Agency's Web site at www.epa.gov/mercury.

Go Nuts With Your Diet

If you've been avoiding nuts for fear of fat, you should probably reconsider: Although nuts are higher in calories because of their fat content, they also are rich in nutrients that may help guard against Alzheimer's. Nuts like almonds, pecans and walnuts contain antioxidants that can protect brain cells from free radical damage.

And although nuts do contain fats, most of the fat is the healthy variety, monounsaturated fat, and can help lower cholesterol. Certain nuts may lower the risk for cancer and reduce blood pressure, too. Eating nuts can also help rein in your appetite, which in turn, can help with weight control.

Limit Your Fats and Cholesterol

It's true that your brain cells are made of fat, but consuming too much fat in your diet poses health hazards. Too much saturated fat and cholesterol clogs the arteries and raises the risk for Alzheimer's, cardiovascular disease, diabetes, and stroke. Common sources of saturated fat include butter, meats, salad dressings, and whole milk dairy products. Food sources of cholesterol include egg yolks, meat, dairy products, and seafood.

Another villainous fat is trans fatty acid, a fat produced during the hydrogenation process that manufacturers use to help extend the shelf life of a food. Processed foods such as crackers, cookies, margarine, cakes, snack foods, fried foods, and fast foods are generally high in trans fatty acids. In general, foods high in fat promote weight gain because gram for gram, fats contain more calories than proteins and carbohydrates. To help lower your fat intake, stick with mono- and polyunsaturated fats, such as olive oil, and practice baking and grilling your foods instead of frying.

Maintain a Healthy Body Weight

At this time, more than two-thirds of the U.S. population is overweight or obese. The rise parallels an increase in the numbers of people with cardiovascular disease and diabetes, which are all problems associated with being overweight. And as the population continues to live longer, being overweight will also play a role in the growing numbers of people who develop Alzheimer's.

Studies have found that people who keep their body weight at a healthy level are generally at lower risk for developing dementia. Lower body weight is also associated with lower cholesterol and blood pressure, two other factors that have been associated with a higher risk for dementia.

Maintaining your weight at a healthy level should continue even as you age. A study in 2003 found that women who were significantly overweight at age 70 were more likely to develop Alzheimer's later on, when they were between the ages of 79 and 88. More specifically, the study defined being overweight as having a high Body Mass Index, a measure of weight in relation to height. In the study, which was done in Sweden, women who had a BMI above 29 were more likely to develop Alzheimer's. A healthy BMI is between 18.5 and 24.9. BMI is calculated by multiplying your weight in pounds by 703. Divide that number by your height in inches, squared (i.e., height x height). A woman who is 5 feet 4 inches, or 64 inches tall and weighs 170 pounds will have a BMI of about 29.

Among people who actually have Alzheimer's or are on the brink of developing it, the problem may be just the opposite—they may experience weight loss. In fact, a 2005 study in the *Archives of Neurology* found that weight loss in elderly Japanese-American men may be associated with dementia. Although the weight loss may not contribute to dementia, it does suggest that weight loss could be a marker of impending dementia and that something is occurring in the parts of the brain that control appetite or metabolism.

If you have Alzheimer's and are having trouble sustaining a healthy weight, talk to your physician or a nutritionist about strategies for eating more and increasing your calorie intake.

Consider Taking Supplements

Certain vitamins, minerals, and herbal supplements have been associated with brain health. Though research on some of the products is mixed, there is some evidence to suggest that these supplements might help boost memory and reduce the risk for dementia.

Gingko Biloba

Extracts from the leaves of the ancient Chinese gingko biloba tree may improve memory and slow the progression of dementia.

Gingko may work by increasing blood flow in the brain and boosting neurotransmitter activity. It also enhances the absorption of glucose, the main source of energy for the brain. Not all studies have demonstrated that gingko boosts memory, but a major clinical trial now underway is examining gingko's effects on the elderly who have Alzheimer's disease.

Vitamin C

Vitamin C is an antioxidant, with the potential for slowing the damage caused by free radicals. Studies suggest that vitamin C ingested through food offers lowers the risk for developing Alzheimer's, but whether a supplement can help is uncertain. Good sources of vitamin C include in the diet include red bell pepper, broccoli, leafy green vegetables, oranges, and strawberries.

B Vitamins

In the body, the B vitamins play numerous roles, including the production of body cells, the production of hemoglobin in the blood, and the production of important body chemicals. In elderly people, the ability to absorb vitamin B12 is often diminished. A deficiency of this vitamin produces symptoms that mimic Alzheimer's.

Researchers now believe that certain B vitamins—namely vitamin B6, folate, and vitamin B12—may play a role in treating Alzheimer's by reducing the levels of homocysteine in the blood. Homocysteine is an amino acid that has been associated with a greater risk for vascular diseases, such as cardiovascular disease, stroke, and Alzheimer's. Damage to the blood vessels caused by elevated levels of homocysteine may raise the risk for Alzheimer's.

The U.S. National Institute on Aging is currently doing a phase III clinical trial to test whether high doses of folate, vitamin B6 and vitamin B12 can slow the rate of cognitive decline in people who have Alzheimer's disease.

Vitamin E

Until recently, many doctors gave Alzheimer's patients vitamin E as part of their treatment regimen. Several studies had suggested that this fat-soluble vitamin could help reduce the risk for dementia. The belief was that vitamin E, which is an anti-oxidant, worked by preventing oxidative stress caused by free radicals, highly reactive molecules that can damage brain cells and promote the development of neurodegenerative diseases like Alzheimer's. One study funded by the National Institutes of Aging, had found that a daily dose of 2,000 IUs of vitamin E offered a modest benefit to participants in moderately severe stages of the disease.

But in January 2005, a study published in the *Annals of Internal Medicine* reported that taking more than 400 international units of vitamin E each day slightly increased a person's risk for dying from all causes. Researchers had analyzed data from nineteen previous clinical trials in which participants took vitamin E for various reasons including the prevention of heart disease and cancer, and the treatment of Alzheimer's disease. In the aftermath of this alarming study, most physicians have stopped prescribing vitamin E to their patients.

GETTING YOUR EXERCISE

For years, you've heard about the virtues of regular exercise—how it maintains weight, staves off cardiovascular disease, diabetes, and other illnesses, and helps maintain muscle strength and aerobic capacity. Research suggests that exercise also has protective benefits for the brain and can help stave off problems such as dementia.

Having Alzheimer's should not mean the end of doing physical activity. In fact, getting your exercise is as important as ever. Regular exercise helps keep muscles strong, promotes better sleep, and can eliminate a bad mood. It may also help lower stress and decrease anxiety. In addition, exercise improves oxygen flow, which can benefit brain cells. And while exercise may not necessarily slow the progression of Alzheimer's, it may help reduce the physical disabilities associated with the disease in later stages.

Among the most interesting studies to support the benefits of exercise in patients with Alzheimer's was one done in Seattle by researchers at the University of Washington. The study, which was published in the *Journal of the American Medical Association* in 2003, looked at the impact of a caregiver-lead exercise program on patients with Alzheimer's and compared it to a group of patients who did not participate in the exercise training.

The study found that patients who were in the exercise program were three times more likely to exercise at least an hour a week and had two-thirds fewer days of restricted activity than those who did not receive the training. Over the next two years, the physical ability of those in the exercise program improved, while those in the other group experienced a deterioration in their abilities. Those who exercised were also less likely to be institutionalized—only 19 percent were placed in nursing homes during the study period compared to fifty percent in the non-exercise group. The authors noted that "improved physical conditioning for patients with Alzheimer's disease may extend their independent mobility and enhance their quality of life despite progression of the disease."

ACTIVITIES YOU CAN DO

The exercise you choose to do doesn't need to be overly strenuous or push you to the brink of exhaustion. It should be just enough to keep you flexible, strong, and to get your heart pumping ever so slightly. It should also be an activity that suits your fitness level and sustains your interest. Exercises that cause injury or bore you are not likely to become a part of your daily routine.

The type of exercises you do will depend largely on the shape you're in and what you were doing before you were diagnosed with Alzheimer's. Among the best is walking. It's easy to do, requires no special equipment beyond a pair of good walking shoes, and doesn't require that you go anywhere special. You can simply don a pair of sneakers and head outdoors for a walk. It's also the least likely exercise to cause injury. You can adapt your walks to suit your fitness level, too. For instance, as you build your stamina, you might consider taking longer walks, going up more hills, or walking faster. And if you choose to walk with a companion or a walking club, you can also savor the social aspects of a good walk. In bad weather, consider walking in a mall or using a treadmill.

But don't feel limited to just taking walks. Other good exercises for people with Alzheimer's include gardening, swimming, water aerobics, and yoga. You may also consider doing tai chi, an ancient Chinese martial art that involves a series of gentle movements and breathing techniques. In one study of adults in later stages of Alzheimer's, researchers found that patients were able to slow the decline of their functional abilities by doing a combination of physical therapy and tai chi, The movements in tai chi are designed to facilitate the flow of energy in your body, but also can create a calming effect and reduce stress.

No matter what you decide to do, the goal is to stay as active as you can for as long as you can. Before starting any exercise program, check with your doctor first and get recommendations about the types of activities you can do and those you should avoid.

When you do start your exercise program, always begin with a gentle warmup and end with a cooldown. Exercise in a safe environment and avoid places with bad lighting, slippery floors, throw rugs, uneven roads, and any other place that could cause you to get hurt. If you have difficulties maintaining balance, exercise near a bar or rail. If standing is difficult, stick with floor exercises. Always discontinue your routine if you experience pain or don't feel well.

KEEP THE BRAIN ACTIVE

You've heard the saying, "Use it or lose it." The saying is often used to refer to body strength, but is just as applicable to intellectual exercises that keep the brain healthy and strong. More and more, researchers are now realizing that keeping the brain active may help stave off the effects of cognitive decline. Whether it can actually prevent Alzheimer's remains uncertain, but it does appear to slow the disease process.

Perhaps the greatest proof of the power of lifelong learning was found in the famous Nun Study. In that study, experts looked at 801 elderly Catholic nuns, priests and brothers from all around the United States. Researchers at the Rush Alzheimer's Center in Chicago looked at how often the nuns engaged in cognitive activities that involve processing information, such as reading the newspaper, reading books, watching television, and going to museums.

After four and a half years, 14 percent of them had developed Alzheimer's. On average, the researchers found, the risk of developing AD was 47 percent lower in people who did these activities the most frequently. Researchers don't know the reasons why, but these activities seemed to protect the brain from cognitive decline. Those who participated in these activities more frequently also had less decline in their working memory. Based on this study, it appears that mentally stimulating activities confers some protective benefits against cognitive decline.

Numerous activities can stimulate the brain. Among the best is reading, which stimulates several parts of the brain and strengthens synapses between neurons. Other mind-bending activities include doing crossword puzzles, writing, playing games, and watching educational television programs. In recent years, numerous people who have early Alzheimer's have started on-line journals and participated in on-line chat rooms, activities that require typing on a keyboard, writing and expressing your thoughts. All these activities can help keep your brain active.

But for someone in the throes of early Alzheimer's, it may be difficult to find the initiative to do these mentally stimulating activities. Rather than find these activities stimulating, people who have early Alzheimer's may find them exhausting and frustrating. They may find it difficult to concentrate or to recall what they've just read or seen. When they attempt these activities, they might become discouraged and frustrated if their efforts are met with failure.

As with other aspects of your life, you may simply have to lower your expectations if you have Alzheimer's. If you've been an avid reader all your life and still want to read, then by all means do so. But don't expect that you'll recall the details of what you've read or that you will have the same concentration skills. Or if you enjoy crossword puzzles, keep doing them. But again, realize that your ability to come up with the right words may not be what it once was. When it comes to mentally stimulating activities, the goal is to use your remaining intellectual powers to the best of your abilities, but not to push yourself to the point of frustration and exhaustion.

GET YOUR SLEEP

Enjoying a good night's sleep may be easier said than done for the person who has early Alzheimer's. Disruptions in sleep are a result of changes in the sleep-wake cycle, which is regulated by the brain. They may also be caused by medications, other medical conditions such as depression, or a bad sleep environment.

To try and ensure good sleep, practice the following:

- Stick to a regular bedtime schedule as much as you can. That means getting out of bed at the same time every morning and going to bed at the same time every night. You should also stick to a schedule for meals and activities throughout the day.

- Avoid drinking or eating anything with caffeine, such as coffee, tea, soda, and chocolate, which can disrupt the sleep-wake cycle, too. You should also avoid drinking alcohol, which can disturb sleep.

- Try to get some regular exercise every day. Even a short walk or some gentle stretches can help. Regular physical activity helps promote sleep.

- Expose yourself to bright light. Being in bright light helps set your circadian rhythm, which orchestrates the timing of your internal bodily functions and will make you alert during the day and more fatigued at night.

- At night, keep your sleep environment dark. Place dark shades on bright windows, and keep shades and curtains drawn. The darkness in the evening also helps establish your circadian rhythm. If you're concerned about falling or tripping, use night lights if necessary.

- Avoid excessive stimulation in the evening hours. Television shows that are too exciting or conversations about heated topics can disrupt sleep. Try reading, taking a bubble bath, or listening to music instead.

- If you suspect that medications are the culprit behind your sleeplessness, consult your physician about changing drugs or altering the dosage.

STAY BUSY

You may not be able to burn the candle at both ends anymore, but keeping active is important for going on with your life, even as you wrestle with the changes imposed by Alzheimer's. There's no need to make drastic changes in your routine at this point. So if you're accustomed to having coffee with a friend every Friday morning, continue doing so. If you have always enjoyed working in your vegetable garden, then by all means, keep tending it. You might also want to continue to do your share of housework and small chores around the house. In some cases, people with early Alzheimer's may even discover new activities and interests that will occupy them.

If you need help performing some of these familiar tasks, don't hesitate to ask. Over time, your abilities may change, and you may not be able to do some of these things as well or you may need to scale back. The key is to adapt the activity to what you can do in the present moment.

JOIN A SUPPORT GROUP

One of the most important things that a person with Alzheimer's and his caregiver can do is to join a support group. Sharing your experiences with others who also have the disease can be a source of enormous comfort. These support groups can also be a source of information, where patients share strategies for coping with Alzheimer's. Support groups can be so vital in the success of your coping with the disease that we will go into them later in another chapter.

CONSIDER VOLUNTEER WORK

If Alzheimer's forces you to give up a job, you might find that you have more time on your hands than you like. Like many retirees, you may want to consider doing some volunteer work. Doing volunteer work allows you to stay active and busy but without the pressure of performing for a boss. It also allows you to stay connected to your community and to contribute something that an organization finds important, which can be reaffirming for someone just diagnosed with a devastating illness like Alzheimer's.

Given that you have early Alzheimer's, you may want to choose your volunteer activities carefully. For instance, if driving is too risky for you, you may want to do something from home like stuffing envelopes or typing up simple documents. Or, if you still have the skills, you may want to make crafts for an upcoming craft fair at your church. Whatever you choose to do, keep in mind that volunteer work is both stimulating for the mind and nourishing for the soul.

CHAPTER SEVEN ❧

Medications for AD

If you have high cholesterol, you have the choice of several different medications to lower your cholesterol. If you have diabetes,
you can choose from a modest list of drugs to tame your blood
glucose control. But if you have Alzheimer's disease, your treatment options are limited to only five medications at this time.

With the numbers of Alzheimer's patients expected to explode
in coming years, researchers across the nation are working furi-
ously to develop a treatment that can delay the progression of the
disease, or prevent it altogether. Researchers, doctors, and families
afflicted by the disease dream of someday finding a cure or a vaccine that can put an end to Alzheimer's. But at this time, the medications we have available can only minimize the cognitive and
behavioral symptoms of the disease.

For people diagnosed in the early stages of Alzheimer's, these
drugs offer at least some hope for an improved quality of life.
Granted, not everyone experiences relief from these medications. Some may need to experiment with several drugs and
dosages before finding the right one. Others may not experience

improvement in their cognitive functioning. Often it requires trial and error to figure out which one, if any, works for you, or whether a combination approach might be better.

CHOLINESTERASE INHIBITORS

Acetylcholine is a chemical messenger in the brain that is involved in the formation of memories, thought, and judgment. It is also involved in controlling muscle contractions and hormone secretion. When certain brain cells transmit messages to other brain cells, acetylcholine is released and then broken down by various enzymes, including one called acetylcholinesterase. The acetylcholine is then recycled and reused.

In the mid 1970s, scientists discovered that in people who have Alzheimer's, levels of acetylcholine in some parts of the brain were dramatically lower than they are in healthy people. That's because the brain cells in these regions are damaged or destroyed, causing levels of acetylcholine to drop. In fact, scientists have established that acetycholine is directly linked to the severity of dementia—the less you have, the worse your dementia.

In the quest for therapies, researchers began looking for drugs that could slow the breakdown of acetylcholine in order to lessen the symptoms of Alzheimer's. The drugs that achieve this effect are known as cholinesterase inhibitors. These medications are used in the early to moderate stages of the disease and have been found to stabilize, even improve cognitive function. In randomized, double-blind, parallel-group clinical trials—considered the gold standard of research protocol—all of them have shown greater efficacy than placebo.

At this time, there remains some controversy regarding the efficacy of these drugs. But with no cure in sight, you may very well consider it worth the risk to take these medications in the hopes that they will help improve your functioning and slow the progression of the disease. If that's the case, be sure to talk it over with your doctor and to tell him about any other medicines you are taking and any preexisting conditions. Experts do know that these drugs should be used with caution in patients who have had cardiac conduction abnormalities, asthma, seizures, active gastrointestinal disease, or in patients taking non-steroidal anti-inflammatory drugs.

DONEPEZIL (ARICEPT)

Approved by the FDA in 1996, donezepil has emerged as the most commonly prescribed cholinesterase inhibitor for the treatment of Alzheimer's. The drug is designed to improve memory and cognition, and help the patient do better performing the activities of daily living.

Although donepezil doesn't cure Alzheimer's, several studies have found it does improve cognitive functioning in some individuals and may delay nursing home placement. In some patients, the drug may demonstrate no effect, and in advanced cases of AD, donepezil may not work at all.

Donepezil is a tablet given once a day, usually at night, at an intial dose of 5 mg. If the drug is well tolerated, the dosage may be increased after four to six weeks to 10 mg. a day.

Side effects from taking donepezil include diarrhea, vomiting, nausea, fatigue, insomnia, and anorexia. In some cases, side effects are mild and diminish with continued use of the drug. In others, these side effects may necessitate discontinuing the medication.

RIVASTIGMINE (EXELON)

Rivastigmine was approved by the FDA in 2000. Like donezepil, it inhibits the action of acetylcholinesterase. But rivastigmine also inhibits butyrylcholinesterase, another enzyme involved in the breakdown of acetylcholine. The drug is used to treat mild to moderate Alzheimer's and has been found to improve cognition and allow greater participation in day-to-day activities.

Rivastigmine is available as a capsule or a liquid. To minimize side effects, such as nausea, the dosage is initially low, about 1.5 mg. twice a day, and increased slowly—no more than once every two weeks—to no more than 12 mg. a day. At higher levels, you are more likely to experience side effects such as upset stomach, vomiting, loss of appetite, weight loss, diarrhea, dizziness, sweating, urinary incontinence, and fatigue.

In patients who do experience side effects, the drug may be discontinued for a few days. Then they may resume taking it again at the same dose or a lower dose. If you do not take it for several days, talk to your doctor before taking it again. Your doctor will probably recommend that you start at the lowest dose.

GALANTAMINE (REMINYL)

Galantamine is the newest cholesterinase inhibitor on the market, and was approved by the FDA in 2001. The drug is available in tablets in 4, 8, or 12 mg. doses. It is recommended that you begin at 4 mg., twice a day. If the drug is well tolerated after four weeks, the dose is usually bumped up to 8 mg. twice a day. And if the drug is still well tolerated after another four weeks, your doctor may recommend that you increase the dosage up to 12 mg. twice a day. The increased dosage should be at your doctor's discretion.

Like the other drugs in this category, you may experience upset stomach, vomiting, loss of appetite, weight loss, diarrhea, dizziness, sweating, urinary incontinence, and fatigue.

In early 2005, the safety of galantamine was called into question after two studies on the drug's effects on mild cognitive impairment found that more patients taking the drug had died than those who were taking a placebo. The "imbalance" in the number of deaths found that out of 2,000 patients, fifteen people taking galantamine died compared with five deaths in the group of people who were not taking it. At the time of this writing, the makers of galantamine, Johnson & Johnson Pharmaceutical Research & Development, were "analyzing additional data from these studies, including information retrieved from subjects who had dropped out of the trials, and is discussing the results with regulatory authorities," according to information on their Web site. Whether the imbalance was a statistical fluke or a bona fide medical concern remains uncertain.

TACRINE (COGNEX)

Cognex was the first cholesterinase inhibitor to receive FDA approval back in 1993. Today the drug is rarely prescribed and no longer marketed because of its link to liver damage.

THE NMDA RECEPTOR ANTAGONIST

Memantine (Namenda) was first approved in Germany in 1982, and has since been used in Europe for the treat of several neurological disorders. In 2003 it was approved by the FDA for the treatment of moderate to severe Alzheimer's. Like the other medications available for AD, memantine does not stop the destruction of Alzheimer's, but can alleviate the symptoms and improve cognitive functioning in some patients.

Memantine is not a cholinesterase inhibitor but rather an N-methyl D-aspartate (NMDA) antagonist that is believed to work by regulating levels of glutamate, a chemical dependent upon glutamate plays a critical role in our abilities to process, store and retrieve information. In healthy people, proper amounts of glutamate trigger receptor channels on the nerve cells called NMDA receptors. NMDA receptors, in turn, allow a controlled amount of calcium to enter a nerve cell, thereby creating an environment that allows for learning and memory. Without enough calcium, the chemical environment of the brain is not appropriate for the proper functions of learning and memory.

But in someone who has Alzheimer's, it is theorized that there is excessive amounts of glutamate. The excess glutamate causes overstimulation of the NMDA receptors, which in turn, allows too much calcium into nerve cells. The excess calcium damages and destroys the nerve cells, leading to the symptoms we see in Alzheimer's. Memantine is believed to work by partially blocking the NMDA receptors and helping maintain normal levels of glutamate thereby preventing neural dysfunction and damage.

Memantine comes in 5 and 10 mg. tablets and is usually taken once or twice a day with or without food. Patients usually start by taking 5 mg and gradually increase to the target dose of 10 mg twice a day by the fourth week. Side effects of the medication may include increased fatigue, dizziness, headache, constipation, and vomiting.

Because its actions differ considerably from those of the cholinesterase inhibitors, memantine may be used alone or in combination with these other medications. In fact, one study found that patients in the moderate to severe stages of Alzheimer's fared better when they took memantine with donepezil than those who took donepezil with a placebo.

HOPE FOR A VACCINE?

Imagine a day when a simple genetic test would reveal that you were at risk for Alzheimer's, then getting a vaccine that would shield you for life from ever developing the disease. The notion of eradicating Alzheimer's with a simple shot, much in the same way that smallpox and rubella have largely been eliminated, is undoubtedly appealing. With a vaccine, you could train the immune system to recognize and attack even the slightest buildup of beta-amyloid plaque, thereby halting the deposits of amyloid and stopping the disease.

Initial results in mice were promising, but when the first vaccines were used in humans, brain inflammation occurred in some of the participants. The makers of the vaccine, Elan Pharmaceuticals, wisely decided to stop the trials. Scientists continued following some of the participants and found that some of those who received the vaccine did experience slower progression of the disease. Upon autopsy, those who had received the vaccines also had less Alzheimer pathology in their brains.

In the aftermath of the Elan experiment, researchers say they have learned a great deal about why the first vaccine may have caused brain inflammation. Recent studies show promise that an approach may be found to avoid the inflammation issue. Scientists have also found that monkeys may provide a valuable animal model for studying Alzheimer's vaccines. In one study, vaccinated monkeys actually developed significant levels of antibodies to beta amyloid. These findings offer hope that someday a vaccine will be developed in the prevention of Alzheimer's.

OTHER MEDICATIONS YOU MIGHT TAKE

Because Alzheimer's is a complex disease, it's no surprise that it can produce myriad symptoms and behavioral problems that may warrant the need for other medications. Among the most troubling behaviors are those known as agitation. In the early stages, agitation may include irritability, anxiety, or depression. Later on, as the disease progresses, it may cause sleep disturbances, delusions, hallucinations, pacing, obsessive-compulsive behaviors, distress, and the uncharacteristic use of bad language.

Agitation may be brought on by Alzheimer's, but it may also be caused by other medical conditions or the use of medications. Sometimes, a patient may become agitated because of a life change such as an abrupt change in living arrangements or the arrival of a new caregiver. In any case, you should discuss your symptoms and concerns with your doctor to try and pinpoint the source.

Sometimes, agitation can be relieved by making minor changes in the environment. Simplifying the routine, creating a safer, less cluttered living space, or providing opportunities for short naps in the day may be all it takes to relieve a person's agitated behavior. But on occasion, you may need medications to get relief.

For the treatment of irritability and depression, your doctor may prescribe these kinds of medications:

- *Selective serotonin reuptake inhibitors (SSRIs)*. These medications work by blocking the removal of serotonin, a neurotransmitter involved in regulating mood, from the gaps between the nerves. Inadequate amounts of serotonin, as well as other neurotransmitters such as dopamine and norepinephrine may cause depression. In recent years, these drugs have become enormously popular as the medication of choice for treating depression. Common drugs include fluoxetine (Prozac), paroxetine (Paxil), escitalopram (Lexapro), and sertraline (Zoloft). Possible side effects include jitteriness, headache, nervousness, insomnia, and sexual problems.
- *Antidepressants that block the reuptake of other brain chemicals*. Some drugs used to treat depression stabilize more than just serotonin and also impact other neurotransmitters in the brain such as norepinephrine and dopamine. Drugs in this loosely organized category include buproprion (Wellbutrin), venlafaxine (Effexor), and mirtazapine (Remeron).
- *Tricyclics*. These drugs are no longer used as first choice treatments for depression, but may be used if other therapies fail. Tricyclics work by restoring chemical imbalances in the brain that can cause depression. Among the drugs in this category are imipramine (Tofranil) and nortriptyline (Aventyl). These medications generally have more side effects than the

SSRIs, including dry mouth, constipation, blurred vision, and they also may affect the heart.

If your agitation produces symptoms of anxiety, restlessness, verbally disruptive behavior, and resistance, your doctor may prescribe an anxiolytic, or anti-anxiety, medication. Two drugs in this category that may be prescribed include lorazepam (Ativan) and buspirone (Buspar).

If you experience hallucinations, delusions, aggression, hostility, and uncooperativeness, you may be given an antipsychotic medication such as olanzapine (Zyprexa) or risperidone (Risperdal). In some cases, your physician may prescribe an anticonvulsant or mood-stabilizing medication that is also used to treat seizures in epileptic patients. Some drugs in this category are divalproex (Depakote) and gabapentin (Neurontin).

SLEEP REMEDIES

In people who have Alzheimer's, sleep disturbances are common. You may have trouble getting to sleep or wake up frequently in the middle of the night. You may awaken earlier than you should. As the disease progresses, the lack of sleep can cause uncontrollable restlessness, and some people may begin to wander. Sleep problems may be exacerbated if you also suffer from depression, restless leg syndrome (an uncontrollable urge to move your legs move at night), or sleep apnea (an abnormal breathing pattern that causes you to stop breathing many times a night). As a result, you may wind up sleeping more than usual or not getting enough sleep.

Resolving your sleep problems often involves establishing a consistent sleep schedule, creating new sleep-inducing habits at bedtime, getting more physical activity, and avoiding foods and beverages that contain stimulants such as caffeine. But if non-drug therapies fail to improve sleep, your doctor may recommend that you try a medication. Medications that help promote sleep include some of those that have already been mentioned for the treatment of other symptoms. Or your doctor may prescribe:

- *Benzodiazepines.* These commonly prescribed drugs are used to cause sedation, induce sleep, relieve anxiety, eliminate muscle spasms, and prevent seizures. Some typically prescribed for people who have trouble getting to sleep include temazepam (Restoril) and lorazepam (Ativan).
- *Nonbenzodiazepines.* These medications are used for the treatment of short-term insomnia and include zolpidem (Ambien) and zaleplon (Sonata). Additionally, the antipsychotics mentioned above may be used for insomnia.

DRUG PRECAUTIONS

Taken correctly, medications can help make it easier for you to live with Alzheimer's disease or any health condition for that matter. But taking medications of any kind should always be done with caution and under a doctor's supervision.

Before taking a drug of any kind, be sure to tell your doctor if you are allergic to any medications. Your doctor should also know about other drugs you are taking. Tell him about every drug, including allergy treatments, and even something as seemingly innocuous as a multivitamin. Some drugs can cause a bad reaction if they're taken with another medication, or even a dietary supplement, and people who have Alzheimer's are often taking more than one medication at a time. That's why it's also helpful to get all your medications from the same pharmacy, where all your records are kept and readily accessible to the pharmacist who is handling a new prescription.

You should always follow your doctor's instructions when taking a medication. Do not increase or decrease a dosage on your own without checking with a doctor first. If you'd like to discontinue a medication because of bad side effects, you should let your doctor know. Some drugs may involve a gradual weaning process rather than an abrupt discontinuation.

Also, in patients who have Alzheimer's, medications may produce unexpected side effects, even weeks after you've first started taking them. For instance, sedating medications such as those used to treat insomnia may cause increased confusion and raise your risk for falling and fractures. Always ask your doctor if a medication can cause side effects, and look for ways to control them. If you're trying a new insomnia medication for example, choose a night when you don't have anywhere to go the next morning, in case you oversleep.

In addition, people who have Alzheimer's need to take extra precautions against overmedicating or forgetting to take a prescribed drug. You and your caregiver should work out a system that ensures you take your medications on time and in the right amounts. You should also know whether a drug needs to be taken with a meal, after a meal, or before a meal, then try to develop a system that makes sure you follow the right protocol.

To guard against mistakes, find out what to do if you do miss a dose. Even people without Alzheimer's can forget to take a pill. Develop a strategy that will help you remember, whether it's post-it notes, a phone call from a friend, or a medicine dispensing box that sets off an alarm when it's time to take a pill.

A FINAL NOTE

While there are no medications to cure you of Alzheimer's or to stop the progression of the disease, there are drugs that can help improve cognition and alleviate some of your symptoms. Using these medications carefully can be a boon to your day-to-day living and make it easier for you to adapt to having Alzheimer's.

As always, the key is to educate yourself, to learn as much as you can about these drugs, their side effects, and potential interactions with other medications. The knowledge will serve you well as you pin down the best treatment regimen for your condition.

CHAPTER EIGHT ✀

Caring for the Caregiver

Few tasks in life are as difficult as that of becoming a caregiver for someone with Alzheimer's. Early on, the job may be mentally exhausting as you struggle to come to terms with the disease, learn to accept your loved one's cognitive decline, and start to juggle the day-to-day logistics of how you will care for this person. As the disease progresses, you may take on more financial and legal responsibilities as well. Gradually, caregiving becomes more physically taxing as your loved one's own physical abilities diminish and his cognitive skills erode even further. Eventually, you will become fully responsible for your loved one's health, safety, and well-being. It's a responsibility no one really wants.

Throughout it all, you will face a cascade of overwhelming emotions. You will feel great depths of sadness and loss as you watch your loved one's personality change and his cognitive, then physical, abilities disintegrate. You will experience anger over the diagnosis and what has become of your loved one and your life. There will be moments of intense frustration over dealing with your loved one's day-to-day changes in personality and behavior.

You may also feel extremely isolated in your daily struggles and overcome with stress as you try to do it all, especially if you're also working a job and/or looking after elderly parents, children, or other family members.

Caring for someone who has Alzheimer's is indeed a life-altering responsibility. The physical, emotional, mental, and financial toll of being a caregiver is increasingly recognized as a serious challenge of the disease. In recent years, support groups have sprung up to specifically address the needs of caregivers. Researchers have begun examining strategies to improve caregiving, as well as ways that the lives of the caregivers can be enhanced through unique counseling techniques or online support services. Experts are also learning that being a caregiver for someone with Alzheimer's can have such an incredible mental and physical impact on the caregiver that it ultimately creates an entire new category of patients in the healthcare system.

If your loved one has just been diagnosed in the early stages of Alzheimer's, you may not be experiencing any of these problems yet. Or if you're lucky and blessed with extreme resilience, you may not ever suffer any consequences from your role as caregiver. But for the vast majority of people who become caregivers, it is a grueling ordeal. Knowing how it might affect your health and well-being can help you anticipate and prepare for the mighty task ahead.

WHO ARE THE CAREGIVERS?

No one ever signed up to become a caregiver for someone with Alzheimer's. And yet, with approximately four million patients in the U.S. and more than half still living at home, there are millions of people serving as caregivers to people who have the disease.

Most caregivers are family members of the person with AD. The majority are spouses, but daughters, daughters-in-law, sons, siblings, and grandchildren are also potential caregivers. In addition, friends, neighbors, and members of a person's faith community may be involved as well.

Different people will experience caregiving in different ways. While some may suffer family conflict, isolation, and tremendous emotional distress, others may experience a renewed sense of purpose or meaning in life. According to the National Institutes of Aging, research has found that being a male spouse, having a preexisting illness, and getting few breaks from the responsibilities of caregiving tend to make caregivers more vulnerable to the physical and emotional stresses of caring for someone with dementia.

THE PHYSICAL IMPACT

Imagine a job that had no vacations and no coffee breaks, a job where you worked alone most of the time and in which you worked twenty-four hours a day. Now imagine that the job gave you total and complete responsibility for the health, safety, and well-being of another person, someone you love and whose personality has morphed into someone you no longer recognize. It's no wonder then, that caring for a loved one with Alzheimer's takes such a toll on the caregiver's health.

According to the Alzheimer's Association, the caregiver of an AD patient has more health problems than other people at his age who are not providing care. The caregivers report 46 percent more physician visits, use 70 percent more prescription drugs, and are three times more likely to become clinically depressed than non-caregiving peers. And according to a study published in the *Journal of the American Medical Association*, caregivers between the ages of 66 and 96 had a risk of dying that is 63 percent higher than that of people the same age who were not caregivers.

Other studies on caregiver health are equally pessimistic:

- A study by researchers at the University of Alabama found that women involved in caregiving produced significantly more cortisol than those who did not, even after other factors that impact cortisol production were taken into account. Cortisol is a hormone released by the adrenal glands when a person is under stress.
- Researchers at the University of California in San Diego looked at fifty-four caregivers of spouses with Alzheimer's and found that the negative impact of caregiving had a direct link to blood coagulation. The researchers concluded that the chronic stress of caregiving for a spouse with Alzheimer's made caregivers vulnerable to excess blood clotting that could lead to heart attacks and other coronary problems.
- A meta-analysis of caregiver health published in the *Psychological Bulletin* of the American Psychological Association, found that caregivers had weaker immune systems in addition to higher stress hormones. Levels of antibodies, which are a measure of the immune system's capacity for defending against viruses, were fifteen percent lower in caregivers than they were in non caregivers. Caregivers also had twenty-three percent higher levels of stress hormones.

THE EMOTIONAL TOLL

Physical ailments are only part of the problem. Because Alzheimer's progresses so slowly, the disease has frequently been called "the long good-bye." And because the days are so long, caregiving for an Alzheimer's patient has been dubbed the thirty-six hour day.

No one understands this better than the caregivers, who are at the forefront of the disease, watching a loved one become sicker and needier as Alzheimer's robs them of their memories, cognitive functions, and eventually, their basic physical functioning. For them, the prolonged farewell is particularly painful and brutal, and frequently produces a constellation of difficult emotions.

Depression

Although caregiving is not necessarily a cause of depression nor a guarantee that you will become depressed, it is not at all unusual for caregivers to become mild or moderately depressed. The fatigue, exhaustion, and demands associated with caregiving can leave even the most resilient person feeling sad.

It should come as no surprise that people who are caring for someone with dementia are twice as likely to develop depression than those caring for someone without dementia. Caregivers of dementia patients are more likely to devote more time and energy to caregiving, experience problems with their jobs, and have less time to devote to things they enjoy and other family members. They're also more likely to experience more family conflicts. Some people are more prone to depression than others. Women, for instance, who make up the majority of Alzheimer's caregivers, are more likely to develop depression than men. But men are less likely to admit they have depression. Men are also more likely to engage in negative behaviors to cope with depression, such as drinking alcohol and overworking. Men may be more likely to seek outside help, but typically have fewer friends to confide in.

Caregivers who frequently suffer from insomnia are also more vulnerable to depression. The constancy of caregiving for someone with Alzheimer's can make a good night's rest difficult to achieve. Over time, the sleep deprivation can bring on depression.

The sadness that accompanies caregiving is so intense that sometimes, even after the loved one is placed in a nursing home or dies, the caregiver may continue to experience symptoms of depression.

Loneliness

It's not unusual to feel isolated in your struggle to come to terms with Alzheimer's. The disease can cut you off from a once active social life as the demands of caregiving slowly begin to eat away at your free time and energy levels. Not surprisingly, studies have found that loneliness is a strong predictor for depression.

Anger and Frustration

Over time, as your loved one begins to lose more and more independence, you may begin to experience feelings of anger and frustration. Your fury may be directed at your loved one, but it may also be turned toward others, including yourself. Anger is also typical because you have no control over your situation.

Changes in Your Routine

As your loved one's cognitive abilities begin their slow decline, you will gradually begin to take on more and more duties. Some of those responsibilities may be new to you and may add to your frustration. And if the person who has Alzheimer's is your spouse, your workload could increase considerably, especially if your loved one was someone who did a lot around the house. Some of the practical changes that you may experience in the early stages of the disease include:

- *Handling money matters.* Even in the early stages of Alzheimer's, the person who is afflicted may no longer be able to handle tasks involving money, like paying bills, balancing a checkbook, or even making a cash payment in a store. For someone unaccustomed to handling the household finances, managing money may be a difficult and unfamiliar task.

- *Adjusting to lost wages.* Another money matter involves the probable loss of family income, especially if the person who has Alzheimer's and the caregiver are both still in the work force. When the person who has the disease is forced to stop working, the household income may be significantly diminished. If the caregiver is forced to cut back on her work hours, then the economic burden becomes even greater. The stress that comes with the loss of income adds another layer of hardship to a situation already taxed by the presence of a difficult illness.

- *Doing more chores.* When Alzheimer's strikes, there is always an adjustment in the division of labor, especially if the disease affects your spouse or someone you live with. For instance, if your wife was the one who did all the cooking and cleaning, you may need to start assuming more household duties. While she may still be able to cook in the early stages of the disease, she may gradually become a hazard in the kitchen. Or if your husband was the resident lawn keeper and gardener, you may need to start mowing the lawn and tending the garden. Assuming new and unfamiliar chores puts yet another burden on the caregiver.

- *Taking the wheel.* Sooner or later, the person who has Alzheimer's has to give up driving. For the caregiver, that means you will need to do all the driving, which typically means also doing all the errands and grocery shopping. It's a good idea now to start getting in the habit of trying to do all your shopping in one trip, or finding ways to reduce the numbers of outings you need to make.

Self-Care = Better Care

Some people instinctively know how to be better caregivers. They know to read up on the disease, to make time for themselves, to seek help and support from every available resource. They do not burden themselves with guilt over taking time to exercise. They make sure to get enough sleep. And they continue making and keeping their own medical appointments, even as they take loved ones to theirs.

But not all people are so good at self-care. Many people have spent a lifetime of putting others' needs before their own. They may pride themselves on doing everything themselves and have difficulties asking others for help, even with minor tasks. Or they may think that no one else will do anything as well as they can.

Now that your loved one has Alzheimer's, such sentiments may only interfere with your ability to provide good care. Knowing as much as you can about the disease and getting the support you need will not only help you cope with the rigors of caring for your loved one; it may also impact your ability to keep your loved one at home. According to the long-running New York University Spouse-Caregiver Intervention Study, caregivers who were given in-depth education, counseling, and support were less likely to place their loved ones in a nursing home than those in the control group who did not receive the intensive support.

In the first year after the study began, eleven caregivers in the treatment group placed their spouses in a nursing home compared to twenty-four caregivers in the control group without the added help. In the long run, caregivers who got the extra assistance were able to keep their loved ones at home an average of 329 days longer than those who did not receive the extra support. Clearly, everyone benefits from the efforts of a savvy caregiver.

One of the good things about getting diagnosed in the early stages of Alzheimer's is that everyone, including the patient, the caregiver, and family members not involved in the day-to-day caregiving, can start to prepare themselves for the challenges ahead before they land at your doorstep. Here are some things that a smart caregiver can do.

BUILD YOUR KNOWLEDGE

Ignorance is not blissful when it comes to a disease like Alzheimer's. The most important thing you can do is to get educated about the disease. The fact you're reading this book shows that you are already making strides in that direction. Anticipating changes in your loved one's symptoms, behaviors, and personality will prepare you to cope with these changes when they come. It will help you better understand some of the more unusual behaviors and personality quirks and help you devise strategies for how to deal with these changes. It will also help you realize that these are the result of the disease, not anything personal that your loved one is doing to insult or attack you. To learn as much as you can:

- *Read up on the disease.* Go to the library and get books on the topic. Check the Internet, which has a wealth of information about the disease. Log on to Web sites like the Alzheimer's Association at www.alz.org, where you can look at newsletters, articles, and press releases about the disease. For more information, see "Resources" on page 229.

- *Find and join a support group.* Learning through the experiences of others, especially those whose loved ones are slightly more advanced than yours is, can help you find the practical advice you need to handle day-to-day matters. Support groups are also a great avenue for locating community resources.

- *Find a doctor who your loved one likes, but also one who will talk to you, the caregiver.* A survey commissioned by the Alzheimer's Association in 2001 found a major communication gap between caregivers and the doctors looking after their loved ones. Among the findings: 57 percent of caregivers said they wanted information about what to expect as the disease progressed, and only 38 percent said they received such information. But 83 percent of physicians said they do provide that kind of information to caregivers. Similar numbers were found in questions regarding medications, recommendations on caregiving, and the advice on helping patients with day-to-day tasks.
- *Get support and information from other sources as well.* Taking care of someone with Alzheimer's requires a wealth of knowledge about numerous topics that range from the legal and financial to the medical and practical. If you can, divvy up those tasks among other family members. Ask your brother the accountant for help with making financial decisions about tax ramifications. Consult a lawyer friend about choosing a durable power of attorney or making up a will. Talk to your sister the physical therapist about finding the best medical care. The idea is not to burden yourself with doing it all, especially if you have family and a circle of friends who can help.

TAKE CARE OF YOURSELF

When you're in the throes of looking after a loved one with Alzheimer's, it's easy to overlook your own needs, especially if you're also holding down a job, taking care of children, or tending to other relatives. But caring for a loved one with Alzheimer's is one of the biggest challenges any person can ever undertake. In order to muster the strength and energy for it, you need to look after yourself, too.

While your loved one may still be self-sufficient in the early stages, there will eventually come a time when his needs become much greater. Knowing what's to come, you should begin now to create habits and routines that will ensure your own care. Keep in mind that if you don't care for yourself, there will be very little you can do for anyone, including your loved one with Alzheimer's.

Minimize Your Stress

We all know someone who bristles at every red light, who taps her feet in long lines, and who complains at the slightest inconvenience. But we also know people who take all these situations in stride and seem to go through life unaffected by events that make others seethe and rage.

The difference lies in how we perceive stressful events. So while it's true that your caregiving situation may be fraught with difficulties, the stress of the situation is also affected by how you perceive it. The key is to try and maintain some perspective, to take lots of deep breaths, and to try to maintain a sense of humor.

The amount of stress you experience is also affected by several other factors, including your relationship with the person receiving the care, your ability to cope with stress in the past, and whether you have support from others, such as siblings, children, or friends. If you voluntarily chose to become the caregiver, you're also less likely to be stressed out than someone who has taken the job out of sheer obligation.

To keep your stress levels in check:

- *Be on the lookout for warning signs.* Are you suffering from sleep problems? Forgetfulness? Irritability. Chances are, you need to take action to relieve the stress before it gets out of hand.
- *Identify your stressors.* Perhaps you have problems asking for help. Maybe you can't get along with your children. Or

perhaps you suffer from feelings of inadequacy. Pinpoint the source of your stress, and devise ways to overcome it.

- *Figure out what you can and can't control.* You can't force your sister to come over and help you care for your mother, but you can change the angry feelings you have about the situation.
- *Do something about it.* Rather than sit back and stew about a stressful situation, take action. For instance, hire someone to come sit with your mother for the afternoon while you do your shopping rather than wait around for your sister. Pursue a hobby, go for a walk, or call a friend to help alleviate your stress. You might also consider taking up meditation or yoga to lower your stress.
- *Give yourself a break.* Once a week, do something just for you. Set aside ten minutes a day, three times a week to take a walk. Go to the mall and shop, if only for an hour. Sit down and watch a favorite sitcom. Knowing you have that bit of time to yourself can sometimes help you endure the more difficult moments.
- *Ask for help.* When someone offers to help out, take them up on it by giving them a specific task. Resist the urge to say, "Thank you, I'm fine, I'll let you know if I need anything." Instead, say something like, "Actually, it would be great if you could make me dinner once this week," or "I would love it if you could drive him to the doctor's on Thursday." Don't expect others to read your mind and know what you need. Only you can tell them exactly what you want.

Get Your Exercise

If you're like most people, you probably had a hard time finding the time to exercise even before you became a caregiver. Now that you're taking care of a loved one with Alzheimer's, exercise may seem like a complete luxury. Truth is, it's not. Regular physical activity should become a necessity, now that someone else is depending on you more than ever.

As we mentioned above, exercise can help relieve stress. But it also helps keep your weight in check, staves off disease, maintains strength and endurance, and boosts your energy. In addition, it promotes better sleep, reduces tension and anxiety, and helps prevent depression.

In the early stages of Alzheimer's, your loved one may even be able to exercise with you. Consider taking a twenty-minute walk three times a day. If you can't create the time, try to work exercise into your routine. Park far away from the entrances of offices and stores. Take the stairs instead of the elevator. Walk to nearby errands and neighbors' houses. Lift weights and stretch while watching TV. The key is to do it regularly.

Eat Well

When you're upset, lonely, and bored, it's easy to reach for a tempting high-fat, sugary treat. If you're depressed, you may have a hard time mustering the energy to prepare a healthy meal. And when you're in the throes of caregiving and juggling other responsibilities, you simply may not have the time to make healthy eating a priority in your life. The result is a diet rich in processed foods, and high-fat takeout meals, none of which promotes good health if eaten in large amounts on a regular basis.

Sticking to a healthy diet is important to your well-being. A well-rounded meal, rich in complex carbohydrates, fruits, vegetables, protein and healthy fats, can help stave off diseases like cardiovascular disease, diabetes, and certain cancers. It can prevent unhealthy weight gain and high cholesterol, high blood pressure, and insulin resistance.

To ensure that you eat well, stock your house with healthy snacks that you can grab and eat in a pinch. Look for simple recipes that don't take a lot of time to prepare. Make meals ahead of time and stash them in the freezer. Try to limit your intake of processed foods like frozen dinners, packaged baked goods, and snacks. Remember that eating well will keep you healthy and give you more energy to care for your loved one.

Get Your Zzzzs

When we're busy, it's easy to put off a good night's rest in order to fold the last of the laundry, pay the bills, and clean the house. But a good night's sleep is critical to someone who is caring for a sick relative. Try to follow the same bedtime routine every night. Get out of bed at the same time every morning and go to bed at the same time every night. Steer clear of substances that can keep you from getting good sleep, such as caffeine and alcohol. Try to get some regular exercise every day. And create a night time routine that will help settle you down, such as watching TV, reading, or taking a bubble bath.

Join a Support Group

No one should endure the task of caregiving alone. Knowing that there are others just like you going through the same trials and tribulations can be enormously comforting and can also provide you with good information. Through these support groups, you can learn about community resources available to Alzheimer's patients and their families. You can also discuss and learn about strategies for coping with certain situations. In addition, most support groups provide a comfortable forum for you to air any emotions you have about caring for someone with Alzheimer's. More information about support groups will be provided in the next chapter.

Work on Your Caregiving Skills

No one ever took classes to become a caregiver for a loved one. It's an unwanted job that falls upon you when a relative gets sick. So it should come as no surprise that you may not have the skills it takes to provide round-the-clock, seven-day-a-week care to someone who has Alzheimer's.

For some people who have may have been trained as nurses, social workers, or counselors, the task may be a little easier. You may have spent years tending to the needs of others, and those job skills will serve you well now. But for others, the job of caregiving may not come easily. It may even prove extraordinarily difficult, especially if you're not a nurturing person by nature.

But that doesn't mean you can't improve the way you handle the task of caregiving. Rather than throw up your hands in frustration, consider this a job that requires new skills and some learning. One of the most important things you can do is to improve the way you communicate with a loved one who has Alzheimer's. Sharpening your ability to relate to your loved one can help make caregiving a lot easier for both of you. Here are some tips from the Family Caregiver Alliance:

- *Set a positive mood for any interaction.* Speak in a pleasant and respectful manner. Use positive facial expressions, tone of voice, and a gentle touch to help convey your message and demonstrate your underlying affection.
- *Get the person's attention.* Limit distractions and noise. Turn off the radio or TV, close the curtains, shut the door, or move to quieter surroundings. Before saying anything, make sure you have her attention. Use eye contact and gentle touches to keep your loved one's attention focused on you.
- *State your message as clearly as you can.* Use simple words and phrases. Speak slowly, distinctly, and in a reassuring tone.

Refrain from raising your voice. If necessary, repeat the message a few times, making sure to use names of people and places instead of pronouns and abbreviations.

- *Keep questions simple and answerable.* Ask one question at a time; yes and no questions work best. Refrain from asking open-ended questions or those that have too many options. If you can, use visual cues and prompts to help clarify the question and guide the response.
- *Listen with your eyes, ears, and heart.* Be patient if your loved one is struggling to come up with the right words. Pay attention to nonverbal cues that may speak more than words.
- *Break down activities into simple steps.* Encourage your loved one to do what he can, and offer gentle reminders as he moves ahead. Help him when he tries to do something that he can no longer manage on his own.
- *When the going gets tough, redirect and distract.* If you sense an emotional meltdown coming, try changing the subject or environment. Let your loved one know that you know he's upset, and suggest a new activity, such as taking a walk.
- *Respond with affection and reassurance.* People who have Alzheimer's often feel confused, anxious, and uncertain of themselves. Don't bother trying to convince them they are wrong. Rather, focus on how the person is feeling—the emotions are still real—and respond with verbal and physical expressions of support, comfort, and reassurance. Holding hands, touching, hugging, and praise is sometimes all the person needs.
- *Remember the good old days.* While recalling what happened an hour ago may be impossible, people with Alzheimer's are able to recall what occurred many years

ago. Remembering old memories is often a soothing and affirming activity.

- *Maintain your sense of humor.* Never laugh at the person who has Alzheimer's, but do use humor whenever you can when you are communicating with them. Chances are, they will laugh right along.

NOT ALL BAD

No one says caregiving is easy. But studies suggest it does have some positive aspects. Many caregivers view it as an opportunity to fulfill a lifelong commitment to a spouse, or a chance to give back to their parents some of the care they received as children. Some caregivers say it has deepened their religious faith, while others report experiencing closer ties with other people, either through new relationships or existing ones.

The good news is, researchers are learning more all the time about the needs of caregivers. Projects like the NYU intervention study and REACH (Resources for Enhancing Alzheimer's Caregiver Health), an initiative by the National Institute on Aging, are uncovering innovative ways to help support caregivers, be it through support groups, family-based interventions, or computer-based information services. For caregivers whose loved ones are in the early stages of Alzheimer's, the additional knowledge can be reassuring.

CHAPTER NINE ❧

Getting the Support You Need

Perhaps you never imagined yourself as the type of person to attend a support group to share your feelings with strangers. Or maybe you used to shudder at the idea of seeking out a social worker or psychological counseling. Maybe you hated to even borrow a cup of sugar from your neighbor. But if you've just learned that you have Alzheimer's, you may start to rethink some of these preconceived notions about yourself. You may realize that you need more support from your friends and family than you ever dreamed you would. You may also find yourself tapping into community resources in a way you never did.

Creating a solid support network is important to people who have Alzheimer's and their families. Having the disease or caring for a person who has it is not something you want to do alone—or should do alone. The love, support, and assistance of others can play a critical role in how well you and your family cope with the disease.

In an ideal situation, the person who has Alzheimer's has not only one primary caregiver, but a whole network of loved ones and friends who can provide emotional support, practical assistance, and routine care. There would be relatives and friends nearby who could help the caregiver with meal preparation, house cleaning, and errands. There'd be people to stop by and stay with the person who has Alzheimer's, so that the caregiver could get regular breaks.

Building that kind of a network may come easily for some families who are physically and emotionally close. Everyone may pitch in without question and lend a hand. But in today's world, where families often live far apart, it may take considerable effort on the part of the patient and the primary caregiver to create such a network. Some families may also have difficulties getting along, and a diagnosis of Alzheimer's may even cause rife and division. For these families, it may mean greater involvement by support groups, community agencies, and other organizations.

The good news is, the numbers of organizations and support groups for people diagnosed in the early stages of Alzheimer's and their families has grown in recent years. As more people are diagnosed in the earlier stages of the disease, the need for more groups that serve them has grown, too. Experts are recognizing that the needs and abilities of people in the early stages of Alzheimer's are considerably different from those in more advanced stages. Nonetheless, people in the early stages of the disease still need support and assistance.

SUPPORT GROUPS

No one who is diagnosed with Alzheimer's is ever obligated to join a support group. Nor is a caregiver. After all, not everyone feels comfortable sharing intimate feelings with a room full of strangers. And some people may find all the support they ever need from their families and friends.

But for many others, joining a support group is one of the best ways for patients and their families to cope with the disease. Being in a support group means being among people who share similar circumstances and who can understand your plight better than others who have not been diagnosed with the disease. Support groups benefit patients and their families on several levels:

- *Education.* Support groups provide members with a forum for exchanging information about the disease and ways to cope with it. Whether it's new research, strategies for dealing with difficult behaviors, or ways to manage new challenges, patients and caregivers learn from one another.
- *Emotional support.* Living with a chronic disease such as Alzheimer's can arouse a host of feelings. Having a support group provides a safe, environment where you can verbalize your thoughts and emotions among others who share those same feelings.
- *Community resources.* Being among other people who have early Alzheimer's and their families can help you learn about resources in the community that may not be well publicized, such as different respite programs. If you're in the early stages, you may find these resources before you actually need them.
- *Camaraderie.* Among the greatest benefits of a support group are the friendships forged through a powerful, common experience. A support group may become a social outlet for patients and their families who may otherwise feel isolated by the disease. People who are living with Alzheimer's may have difficulty relating to old friends, but may enjoy the new friendships made in these groups.

Types of Support Groups
Not all support groups are the same, which is why it may take you some time to find one you are comfortable with and enjoy. Some are primarily educational and may feature guest speakers who discuss

various aspects of the disease. Others focus on emotional support and offer participants the chance to speak. Some groups are lead by professional facilitators such as nurses or social workers, while others are lead by trained group members.

Support groups may also be highly specialized. Some may serve only younger people who have early-onset Alzheimer's. Others may target only those in the early stages of the disease. Still others may be geared only for spouses who are acting as care-givers or for adults or children whose parents have been diagnosed. Participating in a specialized group may help you focus on concerns specific to your situation.

If you'd rather participate in a support group of a less personal nature, you might consider finding one on the Internet. Several organizations have created bulletin boards, chat rooms, and news-groups for people with common concerns to provide information and offer one another support. One of the best sources is the Alzheimer's Association, which has an entire page dedicated to message boards and chat rooms.

To locate a support group, go to the Alzheimer's Association Web site at www.alz.org and look up your local chapter. You might also want to ask your doctor for information about support groups. Other good people to ask include your clergy, social workers, psychologists, and nurses. You might also consult local community centers, services for the aging, churches, synagogues, and assisted-living facilities. Sometimes friends, neighbors, and colleagues can help connect you to a group, too.

If you do decide to join, attend at least a few meetings before deciding that the group is not for you. Sometimes, it takes a while before you feel comfortable with the other members. Over time, the connection may develop as you become more familiar with the other participants. But if you never quite connect, you may consider trying another group.

RESPITE CARE

Support groups aren't the only source of assistance for people who are dealing with Alzheimer's disease. Although you may still be in the early stages of Alzheimer's and be quite functional, there may come a time when your needs—or that of your caregiver—are much greater.

One of the most important sources of assistance is respite care, a temporary source of care for your loved one with Alzheimer's that gives you a break from your job as a caregiver. Some caregivers may feel guilty about seeking help from a respite service. And in these early stages of Alzheimer's, you may not yet have a need for them. But the day may come when you desperately need that break.

For the caregiver, respite care provides a break from the rigors of caregiving. Whether it's a short trip to the supermarket, a chance to get a haircut, or simply a brief visit to the mall, that reprieve may provide a chance to recharge and rejuvenate. After all, most people do not spend all their hours with one person, much less provide that person with constant care and attention.

Respite care can also benefit the person who has Alzheimer's. It gives him a chance to socialize with others living with the disease and to participate in activities that are safe and structured in a secure environment. It's also a chance to experience some independence, if only for a short period. Done outside the home, it's a chance to get outside the confines of your house and to experience a change of scenery. If respite is provided at home, it may be an opportunity to spend time with a new person who can devote all her attention to him.

Respite care may be offered at home or through community organizations or residential facilities. The respite period may last for a few hours, a full day, or overnight. Costs for respite care vary depending on the provider and the arrangement. You may also involve friends and family members as respite providers, assuming they live nearby, and are available and willing to do so.

But for people without family support or the help of friends, there are agencies that can provide respite. In general, there are three kinds of respite care. They are:

- *In-home care.* A trained aide comes to your home and provides different services, depending on your need. Services might include supervision, recreational activities, medical assistance, exercise, grooming, housekeeping, meal preparation, and shopping.
- *Adult day centers.* These centers provide Alzheimer's patients with a place to go for activities, such as arts and crafts, music, discussions, and support groups. For caregivers who are also holding down a job, an adult day center provides a place for their loved ones to go that is safe, structured, and often home-like. Most centers also provide meals and snacks. Costs, hours of service, and weekend availability will vary depending on the center.
- *Residential respite care.* Some residential facilities provide overnight stays for the person who has dementia. The stay may last one night or could go on for several nights, giving the caregiver a chance for an extended reprieve.

Choosing Respite

When it comes time to select a respite service, do your homework. Call the local chapter of the Alzheimer's Association, the Area Agency on the Aging, and other organizations that service the elderly for information on your options. Describe your situation, and tell them what you want. Find one that meets your needs, provides the hours you want, and has the services you would like for your loved one.

Some people may be concerned about the cost of respite care. While it's true that Medicare and most insurance programs do not cover respite care, you may be able to get some financial assistance from a state or federal program such as Medicaid or the U.S. Department of Veterans Affairs.

If it's an in-home aide you're looking for, take the time to interview that person and assess her skills and abilities in working with someone with Alzheimer's. Ask how they might handle various situations. Get references, and find out about her prior experience and training. And trust your instincts. If you don't feel comfortable with someone, ask for another aide. You may need to interview a few before you find one you like.

If you're choosing an adult day center, make sure to stop in first for a meeting with the staff and to see the center itself. Find out the activities and programs they offer, whether they provide meals and snacks, and what the hours are. You should also ask about safety and how they handle emergency situations. If you have the time, arrange to participate in a program.

If it's a residential facility, you'll need to interview the staff, too and make sure the environment is suitable to your loved one's needs. What kinds of activities and programs do they offer? How are medications monitored? How many staff members are available to tend to the residents? How many other residents are there usually? You should also ask for a tour of the facility. Try to assess its cleanliness, the involvement of the staff, and how the residents are doing.

Easing Into Respite

When you involve respite care, it's important to prepare both the aides and staff and your loved one to accept and hopefully embrace, this new arrangement. Tell the aide about your loved one, his background, his preferences, and his quirks. Don't be shy about revealing troubling behaviors that they should know about. Most aides, especially those who have worked with Alzheimer's patients in the past are well aware of unusual behaviors and quirks in people who have dementia.

You also need to explain respite to your loved one. If your loved one is capable, involve him in the decision. But if not, it will be up to you, the caregiver, to find good respite care and to explain it to your loved one. Keep the explanation short and simple, and provide only as much information as is necessary. If you sense resistance, you may want to tell your loved one that the aide is a friend who is helping around the house, and arrange to stick around the first few visits until both people are more comfortable. If he is going to an adult day center, you might say that he is going there to work as a volunteer or to describe it as a social club. By giving it a more positive spin, you may find that your loved one is more willing to go along.

OTHER SOURCES OF SUPPORT

In these early stages, you may not be in dire need of outside support. But you should be aware that there are numerous services available to help you, when the time does come. Among them:

Alzheimer's Association

For anyone who has been diagnosed with Alzheimer's, tapping into the Alzheimer's Association is a must. The association was formed in 1979, when five family support groups got together to discuss the possibility of forming a national organization. A year later, twenty chapters had been formed. Today, the organization is involved in every facet of the disease, including advocacy, education, and research into the prevention and treatment of AD and the quest for a cure. In all, there are now eighty-one chapters and 300 local points of service. The organization hosts an annual Memory Walk in 680 communities across the country.

For people living with the disease, the Alzheimer's Association offers a Contact Center Helpline that operates around the clock. The center provides information, guidance, and support on everything from understanding memory loss to making legal decisions. It also offers referrals to local programs and services and provides assistance with crises. The number is 1-800-272-3900.

In addition, the Alzheimer's Association provides education services, library services, and safety services. To find them on the Internet, go to www.alz.org. Some local chapters also offer services and support that specifically target people with Alzheimer's in the early stages.

National Family Caregiver Support Program

In 2000, the U.S. government passed the Older Americans Act Amendments and established an important new program called the National Family Caregiver Support Program (NFCSP). The program was developed by the Administration on Aging (AoA) of the U.S. Department of Health and Human Services (HHS). The AoA works with a network of national, state, and local groups to provide five basic services for those involved in caregiving:

- Information about available services.
- Assistance in obtaining access to support services.
- Individual counseling, organization of support groups, and caregiver training to help them make decisions and solve problems.
- Respite care for the temporary relief of caregiving duties.
- Supplemental services, on a limited basis, to complement the care provided by caregivers.

The program is eligible to family caregivers who are caring for adults aged 60 and up. In addition, it is available to grandparents and relative caregivers of children under 18 years of age and those affected by mental retardation and developmental disabilities.

Eldercare Locator

Since 1991, the AOA has operated a service called the Eldercare Locator, a national toll-free service that helps connect older adults and their caregivers with local services for seniors. The service is also available online. Eldercare Locator can help you identify services in your area that can assist you with Alzheimer's care.

The toll-free Eldercare Locator service operates Monday through Friday, 9:00 a.m. to 8:00 p.m., Eastern time, and can be reached at 1-800-677-1116. On the Internet, the Web site is located at www.eldercare.gov.

Faith in Action

On a more local level, the Robert Wood Johnson Foundation has an interfaith volunteer caregiving initiative called Faith in Action. The program brings together volunteers from many faiths to work together to care for members of the community who have long-term health needs, such as Alzheimer's. The volunteers come from churches, synagogues, mosques, and other houses of worship, as well as the community at large. Volunteers provide a variety of non-medical assistance with tasks such as picking up groceries, running errands, driving patients to the doctor, friendly visiting, reading, and helping to pay bills.

A FINAL NOTE

No one can tell you the exact kind of help and support you need as you begin to live with Alzheimer's. And certainly, no one can predict the kind of assistance you will need in the future as the disease progresses. But knowing that there are services available to you can be a tremendous relief. The key is knowing when to tap into those resources and how to make them work for you.

CHAPTER TEN ✺

Taking Care of Business

Worrying about your health is only part of the emotional stress created by Alzheimer's disease. Once the reality of having Alzheimer's begins to set in, you may begin to fret about other more practical matters and your future. Who will make decisions for you when you can no longer make them? Who will care for you when your condition worsens? Where will you live when you can no longer remain at home? How will you finance the cost of your care?

Knowing that you have Alzheimer's gives you the opportunity to have a say in these major decisions before you lose the ability to make them. Making some important legal, healthcare, and financial decisions can give you great peace of mind and help minimize the financial impact of your condition on your loved ones.

It's impossible for us to cover all the different legal and financial concerns that may arise in any individual situation. But with help from Manhattan elder law attorney Clifford A. Meirowitz, chairman of the New York County Lawyers Association Elder Law Committee, we can give you some general information and some important topics to contemplate. To obtain more specific information on legal or financial matters, you should contact your local chapter of the Alzheimer's Association, use the "Resources" section beginning on page 229, or consult a financial professional or an elder law attorney.

LEGAL AFFAIRS

Before you got sick, you were probably accustomed to making decisions, big and small, throughout the day. But when someone has Alzheimer's, the ability to make intelligent decisions is increasingly compromised as the disease progresses. Over time, you will gradually lose the ability to make decisions about your medical treatment, your living situation, financial affairs, and other major issues.

It's difficult to know when these cognitive functions disappear, so it's important to make some decisions while you are in the early stages of Alzheimer's and still competent. The key is to plan ahead. Competency means that you are fully aware of what you are doing. To ensure that your wishes are respected and that sound decisions are made, you will need advance directives, legal documents that allow you to state your preferences about treatment and care, and financial decision-making. In making some of these decisions, you may want to consult an elder care attorney, a lawyer who specializes in issues affecting the elderly. Here are three decisions that you should make as soon as possible:

Choose a Durable Power of Attorney

The most important advance directive at your disposal is the durable power of attorney. Durable means that the appointed person, also called an agent or attorney in fact, will act on your behalf when you can no longer make any decisions yourself. Unlike a power of attorney, the durable power of attorney (DPA) continues to have authority over your affairs even after you have lost the capacity for sound decision-making. Appointing a power of attorney is not legally adequate for someone who is dealing with dementia.

Choose your DPA carefully. The DPA is typically a trusted family member who knows you quite well—usually a spouse, a child, or a close relative—and who ultimately becomes fully responsible for all decisions regarding your welfare, including medical and financial matters. It is important to note that the laws governing DPAs vary widely from state to state. In New York, for example, a DPA does not cover medical or healthcare decisions. In New York, you need a healthcare proxy and/or a living will to cover your healthcare decision-making. The key is always to appoint someone who you know will act in your best interests.

In the event that you have no one you completely trust to serve as your DPA, you should consult an attorney. A lawyer can help you find someone who can act as your guardian through the courts.

Making Medical Decisions in Advance

Before you got sick, you probably told your doctor whether you wanted certain medical procedures. But in the later stages of Alzheimer's disease, the ability to make those decisions is severely hampered. That's where healthcare advanced directives come in. Healthcare advanced directives are simple and important legal documents that permit you to plan in advance of a disability that may render you unable to make medical decisions. There are three basic kinds of healthcare advanced directives:

- A healthcare proxy (HCP) is a legal document in which you appoint an agent to make healthcare decisions for you. The proxy you choose should be someone who would make decisions which are consistent with your wishes should you become incapacitated.
- A living will is a legal document in which you express specific directions as to your wishes with respect to extraordinary measures and life-sustaining procedures such as life support.

You may have strong feelings about the use of artificial life-support systems. Perhaps you believe that you should never be placed on these systems and that death should come naturally. Or maybe you believe the opposite, that everything should be done to keep you alive for as along as possible. In any case, you can make those wishes clear by setting up a living will. The living will states your choices for future medical decisions and allows you to legally limit or forgo any life-sustaining measures that you don't want.

- A do not resuscitate order is signed by a physician and directs that cardiopulmonary resuscitation (CPR) not be performed in the event it is required.

Planning ahead by executing healthcare advanced directives is imperative to ensuring that a patient's treatment decisions are followed in the event she becomes unable to express them herself. It is also important to note that you must make your healthcare advanced directives easily accessible to those who may play a role in providing you with care.

Prepare a Will

Many adults today prepare a will once they have children. But if you still haven't made out a will, you should do so now. A will details how your assets will be distributed after your death as well as who will administer your estate. Without a will, state statutes will determine the distribution of your assets.

MONEY MATTERS

The cost of caring for someone with Alzheimer's can be astronomical. Doctor visits, specialized testing, in-home aides, and medications can add tens of thousands of dollars to your medical costs. And if there comes a time when you need to go to a nursing home, those expenses will skyrocket. Trying to get a grasp on these costs may be overwhelming, if not frightening, to the average person.

The key to preventing economic disaster is good planning. By planning for the future and tapping into all your available resources, you can spare your loved ones financial hardship. Here are some guidelines from the Alzheimer's Association:

Talk About Money

It isn't always easy to discuss money matters, even with the people closest to you. But discussing your financial needs and goals with trusted family members now can avoid problems, conflicts, and mistrust in the future.

Choose a Money Manager

Whether it's your spouse, a child or a trusted friend who's a certified public accountant, designate someone to manage your finances when the day comes that you can no longer handle them.

This person will need to know every detail of your financial and legal affairs. Gather your documents and spend a day reviewing them with this person. Important papers include bank and brokerage account statements, wills, living wills, healthcare proxies, durable power of attorney, insurance policies, Social Security payment information, pension and retirement benefit summaries, monthly bills, stock and bond certificates, and any other forms pertaining to money. Inventory your assets, and know the extent of your estate.

Consult a Professional

A financial planner, an elder law lawyer, or estate planning attorney can work with you and your designated money manager to help manage your finances. These professionals can help ensure that your money is properly managed and also identify resources to assist in your Alzheimer's care.

Look for a professional who has solid credentials, work experience, and educational background. If possible, go with someone who is familiar with elder care and terminal illness issues.

Identify Potential Costs

Having Alzheimer's is costly. But determining those expenses ahead of time can help you prepare for the future. Write down a list of all potential expenses, such as health expenses not covered by insurance, legal expenses, and future housing. How much will it cost to go to an adult day care? How much coverage do you have for prescription medications? Begin exploring residential facilities now, too, and start researching ways that you can afford these costs in the future.

Sources of Income

Now that you know the expenses involved, take a look at your financial resources. These might include:

Healthcare Coverage

Most people over the age of 65 are covered by Medicare, the federal health insurance plan operated by the federal government. You may also be eligible for Medicare if you're under the age of 65 and have been on Social Security disability for at least 24 months. Medicare covers inpatient hospital care and a portion of doctors' fees and other medical expenses. It also covers limited skilled nursing care following hospitalization and limited skilled care at home. But it does not cover long-term nursing home care. For more information about Medicare, check out www.medicare.gov.

Other Health Insurance

If you're younger, you may have private insurance, a group employee plan or retiree health coverage. If you switch plans, make sure to find out whether the new policy provides coverage for pre-existing conditions. If you stop working or cut back on your hours, you may be eligible for COBRA, which allows you to pay for continued group health care coverage for up to 18, 29, or 36 months. The coverage may be enough to cover you until you find a new plan or become eligible for Medicare.

Disability Insurance

A worker who is no longer able to work may have disability coverage through an employer. If you bought a personal disability policy, you can obtain benefits paid in the amount you purchased.

Long-Term Care Insurance

If you bought long-term care insurance, you may be covered for expenses in a nursing home or other extended-care facility. It also may cover home health care, assisted living facility, and adult day care costs. It is essential to buy sufficient coverage, but long-term care insurance is very expensive and is generally not available to people who have been diagnosed with Alzheimer's.

Life Insurance

You may be able to borrow from a policy's cash value or use a portion of the death benefits to pay for long-term care expenses. Some policies may offer "accelerated death benefits," in which a portion of the death benefits are paid before death if you're expected to live for only six to twelve months.

Viatical Settlements

In the later stages of Alzheimer's, you may also consider a viatical settlement. A viatical settlement allows a terminally ill person to reap the benefits of his or her life insurance policy while he is still alive by selling an existing life insurance policy to a third party in return for a percentage of the face value of the policy, which is paid immediately. The buyer purchases the policy, or a portion of it, at a price that is less than the death benefit of the policy. When the seller dies, the buyer collects the death benefits.

For the buyer, viatical settlements are high-risk investments that allow them to invest in another person's life insurance policy. If the seller dies before the estimated life expectancy, the buyer may receive a higher return. But if the seller lives longer than expected, the buyer will receive a lower return. If the person lives long enough that you have to pay additional premiums to maintain the policy, a viatical settlement could become a financial liability.

For the seller, a viatical settlement is a source of tax-free income. For more information about viatical settlements, contact the Viatical and Life Settlement Association of America at 407-894-3797 or online at www.viatical.org.

EMPLOYMENT

Whether you can work depends on your current health and the type of job you do. You may need to make some changes such as cutting back hours or doing less demanding tasks to adapt your work situation to your health. Keep in mind that the American with Disabilities Act offers some protection to people who have Alzheimer's disease. Companies with fifteen or more employees must make "reasonable" accommodations for job applicants with physical or mental disabilities. You can also talk to your employer about benefits such as paid sick leave or other short-term disability benefits.

Retirement Benefits

Money you've saved through your individual retirement accounts, annuities, and your pension plan can provide income, even if you haven't reached retirement age. You can even withdraw money from your IRA or employee-funded retirement plan before age 59½ without paying the ten percent early withdrawal penalty. But you will still have to pay income tax on your withdrawals. So if you're planning to tap into your IRA or employee-funded retirement plan, try to wait until after you leave your job, when you'll be in a lower income-tax bracket.

Personal Savings, Investments, and Personal Property
These include stocks, bonds, mutual funds, savings accounts, certificates of deposit, real estate, and personal property such as artwork, jewelry or collectibles. Before selling assets, consult a financial advisor or tax specialist about tax ramifications.

Your Home
Tapping into the equity you've built up in your home can also provide a source of income. You may consider selling your home and investing the money.

Reverse Mortgages
If you own a single-family home and own it outright, you may consider a reverse mortgage, a type of home equity loan for someone over the age of 62. A reverse mortgage allows you to convert some of the home equity into cash without requiring you to sell your home. As the homeowner, you use your home as collateral against the loan, which is paid to you in a lump sum or periodic payments. The amount you can borrow is based upon your age, your current home equity and the lender's interest rate. But the amount you can borrow is always less than the value of the home.

The loan is not paid back until you die, the home is sold, or you permanently move away. The money you receive is not taxable, and for people who are in the advanced stages of Alzheimer's, it may finance the cost of long-term nursing home care.

Government Assistance

For people who meet certain eligibility requirements, there may be monetary assistance from the government. These programs include:

Social Security Disability Income

People under age 65 may qualify for Social Security Disability Income (SSDI). In order to qualify, you must prove that you can no longer work or that the condition will last at least a year or that it will result in death. Your family members may also be eligible to receive SSDI benefits.

Don't wait to file for SSDI benefits. Although benefits aren't paid until the sixth full month of disability, the Social Security Administration is often slow in deciding whether to approve a claim. Often, an applicant is initially rejected, in which case you'll need to file an appeal. After receiving SSDI benefits for at least 24 months, you will qualify for Medicare.

Supplemental Security Income

People who are aged 65 or older, disabled or blind, and who have very limited income and assets may be eligible to receive Supplemental Security Income (SSI). In order to receive SSI, you must meet the SSA's definition of disability. Again, don't wait to apply for benefits. Payments start as soon as you're approved.

For more information on both SSDI and SSI, contact the Social Security Administration at 1-800-772-1213 or visit the Web site at www.ssa.gov.

Medicaid

For people at very low income and resource levels or those who have exhausted their resources and are in need of long-term care, Medicaid is a possible source of assistance. Most Medicaid dollars go toward nursing home care, but not all nursing homes accept Medicaid. In most states, Medicaid will also pay for hospice care for qualified persons. In any case, Medicaid planning is complex, case specific, and there are variations from state to state as to what is permissible. There is also a tremendous amount of misinformation regarding Medicaid planning.

People who are eligible for SSI are usually eligible for Medicaid. However, those who do not receive SSI can qualify if their income and assets are below a certain amount, which is determined individually by each state. Although Medicaid is a government program designed for poor people, the transfer of assets allows middle class people to access Medicaid, too. But before you start giving away all your assets to loved ones, check with a legal or financial advisor who is well versed on the laws governing the transfer of assets. For instance, anything you give away up to three years before applying for Medicaid is scrutinized by the government. You may also face several legal or tax issues.

Transfer of asset rules are extremely complex, and there are many variations from state-to-state. Some rules protect middle class people by assisting them in preserving assets and still enabling them to obtain the care they need through Medicaid. In New York State the rules governing transfers with respect to nursing home Medicaid or home care Medicaid are very different. There are also special Medicaid rules that protect community spouses as well as disabled children.

For more information on Medicaid, contact your state or county human services or social services department.

Veteran's Benefits

Veterans of war may qualify for government assistance. But these benefits are changing and the number of veteran's medical facilities is declining. For more information, contact the Department of Veterans Affairs at 1-800-733-8387.

Other Public Assistance

Some states have state-funding available for long-term care, as well as adult day care and respite care. To find out more, contact your local Alzheimer's Association, local or county agencies on aging, or the state department or council on aging.

If you think you might be missing out on programs, check out BenefitsCheckUp, a service of the National Council on Aging that is available on the Internet. BenefitsCheckUp screens for federal, state, and some local private and public health benefits for adults aged 55 and up. It contains more than 1,200 different programs from all fifty states and has an average of fifty to seventy programs available per state.

The service also provides descriptions of the programs, contacts for additional information, and materials to help you apply for each program. These programs may help you pay for housing, prescription drugs, health care, utilities, and other essential items or services. To find out if you might qualify, go to www. benefitscheckup.org and fill out the simple questionnaire. The online service is free and confidential.

MAKING FUTURE LIVING ARRANGEMENTS

Having Alzheimer's doesn't guarantee that you'll move to a nursing home someday, but it certainly does increase the odds. As the disease progresses, you may begin to experience wandering and exhibit behaviors that will become increasingly difficult for your caregiver to manage. You may also require greater physical care than your caregiver can provide.

In any case, having Alzheimer's does mean you will probably have to move someday. In some cases, you may need to move closer to other family members who can assist in your care. In others, a spousal caregiver may opt to move to a smaller home.

For some people, there may be a need to find living arrangements that provide round-the-clock care. Keep in mind too, that as your needs change, so too may your need for different living arrangements. Below are the types of housing available.

Retirement Housing

For people who can live independently and have few health concerns, retirement housing is a viable option. These communities, which are also called senior apartments or senior living facilities, provide small studios or apartments that are equipped with cooking facilities. There may also be a common dining area or a community room for socializing. Some homes may also provide activities, some housekeeping, and a variety of activities. But these facilities do not provide health and medical care on the premises. As a result, they are not well suited for people in the more advanced stages of Alzheimer's. They may however, be suitable for people in the early stages of the disease who want to live in a smaller home.

Assisted Living

These types of facilities, also called board and care, group homes, community-based residential facilities, or foster homes, can vary a great deal in terms of what they offer. They are best suited to people who can live somewhat independently but still need some assistance.

Assisted living facilities provide a room that may be private or shared, three meals a day, and in some cases, a small kitchenette. The places are generally staffed twenty-four hours a day, but the staff may or may not be trained to care for people with dementia, and the amount of care will vary. The facilities also provide structured activities, and may also offer laundry, transportation, and help with medication. These homes may be most appropriate for people in the early to middle stages of Alzheimer's.

Nursing Homes

These settings are also known as skilled nursing facilities or health and rehabilitation centers. Nursing homes offer health care around the clock. Some may even feature special units just for the care of people who have dementia.

Residents typically live in a room with a bathroom and may share the room with another person. There are also common rooms for residents to gather. All activities and care are closely monitored and supervised by trained staff. For instance, a registered dietitian supervises meal preparation, and a licensed nurse provides medical care. The staff is generally trained to address the residents' medical, spiritual, and recreational needs.

These facilities are best suited for people in the middle, late, and end stages of Alzheimer's, though they may also benefit someone in the early stages if there are other medical needs involved.

Continuing Care Retirement Communities

Making the decision to live at a continuing care retirement community (CCRC) is typically considered a once-in-a-lifetime choice. These facilities, which are sometimes called life care communities, feature large campuses that provide all the different types of housing described above. So the campus will include residents who live independently, as well as those requiring some assistance and those who need skilled nursing around the clock. Residents move from one facility to another as their needs change. These facilities are often high-priced and may not be available to people with more modest incomes.

CHOOSING A FACILITY

It's best to start considering the choice of a facility before you actually need to move in. The extra time will let you consider your options and help you determine which one is best suited to your needs. The most important considerations are the amount of care required and the atmosphere the patient prefers. According to the Alzheimer's Association, there are several questions you should consider:

- Do you need twenty-four hour supervision?
- What are some characteristics of the person with Alzheimer's that may require special skills of the staff who care for him?
- Does the person with Alzheimer's need help taking medications?
- Do you prefer a private or a shared room?
- How much and what type of social activity do you want from the facility?
- Do you want a facility that cares only for people with dementia?
- What types of meals are required? Do all meals need to be prepared by someone else?
- How will costs be covered?

AFFORDING THE CARE

The cost of living in these types of housing can be high. Retirement homes are generally paid for only with your own money. With assisted living, you may be able to get some help from insurance and Medicaid, though Medicaid varies from state to state. Nursing home costs may be paid for through a combination of private funds, Medicaid, private insurance, and some limited help from Medicare. Early, careful planning for a potential stay in a long-term care facility, either through the purchase of long-term care insurance or through Medicaid planning, can help you meet these costs and save substantial assets, while giving everyone involved peace of mind.

A FINAL NOTE

It isn't easy for people to contemplate some of these issues, especially if they're already struggling with the early symptoms of Alzheimer's. But making some of these decisions before you're in the latter stages of the disease can be reassuring. Even if you cannot predict the course of the disease or what your needs will be in the future, you will have at least made your wishes known and discussed them with your family.

Note: Clifford A. Meirowitz is chair of the New York County Lawyers Association Elder Law Committee, a member of the National Academy of Elder Law Attorneys, the New York State Bar Association Elder Law Section's Executive Committee, and an adjunct assistant professor at New York University's School of Continuing and Professional Studies.

CHAPTER ELEVEN ✀

What Does the Future Hold?

It's been a century since Alois Alzheimer first spotted the plaques and tangles inside the brain of his patient, Auguste D. Our understanding of the disease that bears his name has since grown considerably, much of it in recent decades. But even as scientists around the world scrutinize the various aspects of this baffling disease, myriad mysteries remain. What exactly is the cause of Alzheimer's? Which comes first, the plaques or the tangles? How can we diagnosis it better and earlier, in the stages when people seem to respond better to treatments? What can we do to treat the disease and to slow its progression? And dare we even begin to dream of the day when we can cure Alzheimer's and spare millions of people from the ravages of this disease?

The quest to answer these questions has intensified in recent years as baby boomers gradually enter their mid 60s. At the current rate, experts predict that by the year 2030—when the entire baby boomer generation will be over the age of 65—the numbers of people with Alzheimer's will increase to 7.7 million from its current figure of 4 million. By the year 2050, those numbers could be as high as 13.2 million. With the current cost of caring for people with Alzheimer's estimated between $50 billion to $100 billion, the future costs look ominous—unless the disease can be delayed, prevented, or cured.

With the amount of research now going on, scientists are optimistic that something will happen to slow the trend. Federal funding for Alzheimer's research reached an all-time high in 2004 of $679 million, according to the Alzheimer's Association. A search for "Alzheimer's" on the search engine at www.clinicaltrials.gov, the federal government's Web site on current clinical trials, turned up fifty-four studies alone. The energy and effort being applied to a better understanding of this disease is clearly reaching a fever pitch. In this chapter, we will examine some of the current research that is giving hope to families and patients around the world afflicted by Alzheimer's.

PINPOINTING THE GENES

Figuring out what sets the disease process in motion is one of the mysteries about Alzheimer's that has puzzled scientists for years. Studies have demonstrated that genetics play a role in the disease. For instance, we already know that people who have early-onset Alzheimer's tend to have a strong family history for the disease. Scientists have discovered that people who have early-onset AD have mutations—unexpected changes in a single gene or in sections of chromosomes—in one of three genes. Meanwhile those with late-onset AD were likely to carry a variant of a gene called apolipoprotein E epsilon-4, or APOE-4.

Experts believe that like many other diseases, Alzheimer's develops from a complicated mix of genetic factors and environmental influences. Identifying the genetic risk factors could help predict an individual's risk for developing Alzheimer's. Genetics could also help researchers develop new drugs to slow the course of the disease.

To identify the genes that cause AD, the National Institute on Aging is collecting genetic material from families with several members who have late-onset Alzheimer's, the kind that develops after age 60. The NIA and the National Alzheimer's Association are working with investigators at Indiana University's National Cell Repository for Alzheimer's Disease and Columbia University. The Alzheimer's Disease Genetics Study, as the study is formally called, will include information on 1,000 families.

Genetics are only part of the answer. Not everyone who has a family member with AD will get Alzheimer's, and not everyone who has AD can always identify a relative who had the disease. Figuring out what puts one gene carrier at risk while another is free of disease is another avenue of research.

GETTING AN EARLIER DIAGNOSIS

Experts believe that the biological processes underlying the development of Alzheimer's start years before any symptoms are apparent. They also know that early diagnosis offers the greatest hope for preventing or delaying the disease. But how do we know that someone is in the process of developing Alzheimer's? What are the biological changes? Several studies are providing information that experts hope will lead to new diagnostic tools that will allow earlier detection of Alzheimer's.

Nano-sized Markers

One type of technology that offers hope for an earlier diagnosis is nanoscale technology. Imagine dividing up a human hair into 50,000 parts on its diameter. Or dividing up a meter into a billion parts. That's the size of a nanometer, which is a unit of measure some scientists are working with to pinpoint a protein associated with Alzheimer's.

Using a technology called bio-barcode amplification, researchers at Northwestern University and Rush University Medical Center were able to measure the presence of a protein called amyloid β-diffusible ligands, or ADDLs, in cerebrospinal fluid. Research has found that ADDLs appear in the earliest stages of Alzheimer's before symptoms become apparent. ADDLs are only five nanometers wide and present in the cerebrospinal fluid at a very low concentration, making it hard to detect with conventional technology such as enzyme-linked immunoassays (ELISA) tests which are used to detect the presence of antibodies to make a diagnosis.

In a study, the researchers measured ADDL concentrations in thirty people. The concentration of ADDL was consistently higher in people diagnosed with Alzheimer's than in those without the disease.

The bio-barcode technology offers hope that Alzheimer's could be detected in its earliest stages, when treatments and preventive strategies might be most effective.

According to Chad Mirkin, one of the researchers at the Northwestern University Department of Chemistry and Institute for Nanotechnology: "This study is a major step forward in identifying a routine diagnostic tool for Alzheimer's disease, and it validates our hypothesis that there are many biomarkers for disease that go under the radar of conventional diagnostic tools. The extraordinary sensitivity of the bar code assay has a chance to change the way the medical community thinks about molecular diagnostics and the markers they consider for many types of diseases."

Adds colleague William Klein of the Northwestern University Institute for Neuroscience: "It's a good bet that the very earliest stage of AD memory loss begins when ADDLs attack key synapses in the brain. We predicted some of these ADDLs would leak into the cerebrospinal fluid, but until now we couldn't detect them.

Thanks to the extraordinary sensitivity of the BCA, it's been possible to validate the prediction, and maybe even set the stage for creating the first clinical lab test for Alzheimer's disease."

A Five-Year Plan

In another effort to identify better diagnostic tools, the National Institute on Aging has joined together with other federal agencies, private companies and organizations to launch a $60 million, five-year effort called the Alzheimer's Disease Neuroimaging Initiative.

The study is an attempt to find changes in the brain that suggest the development of Alzheimer's and can be detected by neuroimaging techniques such as serial magnetic resonance imaging (MRI) and positron emission tomography (PET). Prior studies show that PET scans can reveal that people with Alzheimer's metabolize glucose at a slower rate in certain parts of their brain than people without the disease. Scientists will also be examining other biological markers for clues such as cerebrospinal fluid, urine, and blood. The 800 participants in the study will be cognitively normal, have MCI, or be in the early stages of AD. Researchers will track their progress over two to three years.

A Special Compound

As of now, the only way to confirm a diagnosis of Alzheimer's is at death, when an autopsy can reveal the telltale plaques and tangles that invade a brain afflicted with AD. Scientists at the University of Pittsburgh Medical Center however, are perfecting a compound that will enable doctors to detect the presence of Alzheimer's in someone's brain while the patient is still alive.

The substance is being called Pittsburgh Compound B. By injecting it into patients, doctors will be able to confirm a person has Alzheimer's and would eliminate some of the guess work involved in making a diagnosis. Perhaps even more important, the compound will help identify people at risk for the disease years before symptoms are evident. Experts know that brain changes may occur as much as thirty years before symptoms or signs emerge. Given that knowledge, patients may be able to start treatment early and prevent or delay symptoms of Alzheimer's.

Pittsburgh Compound B (PIB) is designed to travel through the bloodstream, enter the brain, and attach itself to beta-amyloid deposits. PIB can then be detected by positron emission tomography (PET) scans. In a PET scan of the brain, areas with the greatest concentration of beta-amyloid should appear red and the area with no beta-amyloid should be blue.

Compound B may also have major implications in the development of drugs for the treatment of Alzheimer's. With the use of Compound B, researchers will be able to assess and actually see the effectiveness of new medications designed to reduce amyloid deposits.

Scientists are still in the process of perfecting the substance. Many people who do not have Alzheimer's, for instance, still have some amyloid in their brains. A compound that can distinguish that kind of amyloid from the destructive variety in Alzheimer's will be important to identifying patients who have the disease.

TREATING ALZHEIMER'S

The quest for medications beyond the five currently approved by the FDA is ongoing, rigorous, and intense. It appears to be a matter of time before new therapies are approved. These are just a few of the drugs now being studied:

Alzhemed

The plaques inside the brain of a person with Alzheimer's are a complex mix of proteins, remnants of neurons, and a substance called beta amyloid, a soluble protein fragment cleaved from a larger protein called amyloid precursor protein. When these beta amyloid fragments bind together, they form the plaques that are a hallmark of Alzheimer's. Some studies suggest that beta amyloid may be the root cause of Alzheimer's, a finding that has spurred some biotech and pharmaceutical companies to focus their energies on finding treatments that interfere with the buildup of beta amyloid. If successful, these medications would be the first disease-modifying drugs that could potentially stabilize the course of the disease and even halt its progression.

In the summer of 2004, Neurochem Inc., the company that is testing Alzhemed, launched the phase III trial of Alzhemed, an experimental drug that may interfere with the disease process in the early stages of Alzheimer's.

Alzhemed works by binding to beta amyloid in the brain before plaques can form. It also helps to remove beta amyloid from the brain and blocks the inflammatory process associated with amyloid buildup in the disease process. Earlier studies found that patients who received the highest doses of Alzhemed were able to sustain, even improve, their scores on cognitive tests, while those who received a placebo experienced a decline. Studies so far have also found that the drug is safe and well-tolerated.

Leuprolide

As a hormone medication, leuprolide is prescribed to men who have prostate cancer, and women who have endometriosis or uterine fibroids. Leuprolide belongs to a class of drugs known as gonadotropin-releasing (LH-RH) hormone analogs. These drugs work by stopping the production of testosterone in men and estrogen in females, hormones that stimulate the growth of diseased cells involved in prostate cancer and endometriosis.

Scientists at Voyager Pharmaceuticals are wondering whether leuprolide may also help slow the progress of Alzheimer's and improve the cognitive function of people with AD. People who have Alzheimer's have elevated levels of hormones known as gonadotropins, hormones that some experts believe are linked to the breakdown of neuron function.

Studies are now underway to examine the effect of leuprolide on men with mild to moderate Alzheimer's disease and whether it can improve cognitive function and slow the disease.

Ampalex

Glutamate is an amino acid and chemical messenger released by brain cells that acts to excite other cells. It plays a pivotal role in information processing, storage, and memory. To do that, glutamate attaches to special receptor cells called AMPA (alpha-amino-2, 3-dihydro-5 methyl 3-oxo-4-isoxazolepropanoic acid) receptors. In people who have Alzheimer's, the brain cells that release glutamate are damaged, so that levels of glutamate are excessive or deficient. Inadequate amounts of glutamate has a negative impact on learning and memory.

Ampalex acts to compensate for that deficit by enhancing the ability of AMPA receptors to attach to glutamate. Early studies have found that Ampalex, also called CX516, enhanced learning and memory in healthy young and elderly adults. Studies are now underway to see whether Ampalex, or CX516, can improve the symptoms of Alzheimer's and be safely tolerated.

Neramexane

Another experimental drug that acts on glutamate is neramexane, an N-methyl-D-aspartate (NMDA) receptor antagonist. NMDA receptor antagonists work by regulating the activity of glutamate, which is involved in information processing, storage, and retrieval. Glutamate triggers NMDA receptors to allow a controlled amount of calcium to flow into a nerve cell, creating the chemical environment required for information storage. Too much gluta- mate overstimulates NMDA receptors to allow too much calcium into nerve cells, which destroys and kills the nerve cells. Nera- mexane may guard against excess glutamate by partially blocking NMDA receptors.

If approved, neramexane would join memantine (Namenda) as the second drug in this category approved for the treatment of Alzheimer's.

SGS742

GABA, which stands for gamma-aminobutyric acid, is a chemical messenger in the brain that relays information back and forth from the sensory organs such as the eyes back to the brain. Scien- tists have found that not enough GABA can lead to the cognitive decline associated with Alzheimer's.

Saegis Pharmaceuticals is currently testing a drug known as SGS742, a GABA receptor antagonist that binds to the receptors of GABA, which would then keep more GABA in the brain. Earlier clinical trials have shown that the drug improves attention and memory. SGS742 has also been found to improve learning in mice, rats, primates, and humans.

AN ANTI-EPILEPTIC DRUG FOR ALZHEIMER'S

For years, doctors have prescribed an anticonvulsant medication called Valproate for the treatment of seizures in epilepsy. The drug has also been used to treat the manic phase of bipolar disorder and to help prevent migraine headaches. Now, scientists are wonder- ing if Valproate may lessen symptoms of agitation in Alzheimer's and slow the cognitive decline associated with the disease.

The National Institutes of Health has launched a $10 mil- lion multi-center study to answer that question. The study will also examine whether Valproate can improve memory and daily functioning and provide protective benefits of neurological functioning. Unlike most experimental treatments that are focused on beta amyloid, this study will examine a drug's potential to block neurofibrillary tangles, the other hallmark of Alzheimer's, which are created by chemical changes in a protein called tau. Early studies show that the drug may work by interfering with molecular events that lead to the progression of Alzheimer's.

PREVENTING PLAQUE FORMATION

Rather than wait for the plaques to form and to then work on reducing them, some companies are aiming to prevent their formation at all. Researchers believe that by inhibiting certain enzymes involved in plaque formation, Alzheimer's disease could be effectively blocked. The two enzymes under scrutiny are gamma secretase and beta secretase, which is also called BACE1. Beta-secretase and gamma-secretase are responsible for cleaving amyloid precursor protein (APP), which leads to the production of beta amyloid. Scientists believe that inhibiting these enzymes might reduce the amount of beta amyloid in the brains of people with Alzheimer's, which might then slow the progression of the disease. But these enzymes are also involved in other bodily processes, which could cause complications.

CAN NSAIDS STOP THE DECLINE?

Ever since the discovery of indomethacin in 1956, doctors and patients alike have turned to non-steroidal anti-inflammatory drugs for the relief of pain and swelling, and the reduction of fever. In fact, today, more than 20 million Americans regularly use an NSAID.

In recent years, scientists have begun to question whether NSAIDs may have a role in the treatment and prevention of Alzheimer's. Long-term population studies have suggested that people who take NSAIDs for arthritis are at reduced risk for developing Alzheimer's. Of particular interest is a drug called flurbiprofen (Flurizan), which was derived from a different formulation of a drug called Ansaid. As one of the weaker NSAIDs, Ansaid has been used to treat arthritis.

In January 2005, Myriad Genetics announced plans to begin a phase III clinical trial, nine months ahead of schedule. The trial, which will be conducted on about 750 patients with mild to moderate Alzheimer's, will determine whether Flurizan can alter the course of the disease and slow the cognitive decline. Participants will be randomly assigned to receive 400 or 800 milligrams of Flurizan twice daily or a placebo. In earlier studies, Flurizan was found to reduce beta amyloid, the protein fragments believed to be the culprit behind the devastating plaques that damage the brain in Alzheimer's.

According to the Alzheimer's Association, several research questions still need to be addressed regarding the use of NSAIDs. What mechanisms of NSAIDs are relevant to AD? Which of the currently approved NSAIDS merit further research? Do some NSAIDS help prevent dementia? Can some NSAIDs treat dementia? Is inflammation in the brain an appropriate target for the treatment or prevention of Alzheimer's? And, are new drugs needed for targeting inflammation?

DO HERBAL SUPPLEMENTS AND VITAMINS HAVE A ROLE?
The use of herbal remedies and vitamins to tame medical conditions has gained popularity in recent decades, thanks in large part to an overall trend toward more natural therapies. Not surprisingly then, researchers are looking at some herbal remedies and vitamins to see if they can play a role in slowing or preventing Alzheimer's. Among them:

Huperzine A
Huperzine A is an herbal supplement derived from the plant Huperzia serrata. In China, it has been used for centuries as a

treatment for swelling, fever, and blood disorders. Recent clinical trials in China have reportedly shown that huperzine can also benefit people with Alzheimer's disease.

Intrigued, the National Institute on Aging (NIA) has launched a clinical trial of huperzine A as a treatment for mild to moderate Alzheimer's disease. This NIA study, which will involve 150 patients, will be the first U.S. clinical trial comparing a standardized preparation of huperzine with a placebo.

Experts believe that Huperzine A functions much like cholestinerase inhibitors such as Reminyl, Exelon, and Aricept. These drugs work by inhibiting an enzyme called acetylcholestinerase and slowing the breakdown of acetylcholine, a neurotransmitter involved in the formation of memories, thoughts, and judgment.

Gingko Biloba

Gingko biloba is an herbal remedy that comes from an ancient tree in China. Extracts from the leaves of the tree may improve memory, and slow the progression of dementia. Gingko works by increasing blood flow in the brain and boosting neurotransmitter activity.

To determine its effects, the National Center for Complementary and Alternative Medicine (NCCAM) is conducting a phase III clinical trial. Participants, who are all at least 75 years old, are being given 240 mg. a day to see whether gingko biloba decreases the incidence of dementia, and specifically Alzheimer's disease (AD). It will also measure whether the supplement can slow cognitive decline and functional disability, reduce the incidence of cardiovascular disease, and decrease total mortality.

The B vitamins

In people who have Alzheimer's disease, blood levels of an amino acid called homocysteine are elevated. Experts know that homocysteine levels can be reduced by high dose treatments of vitamins B6, B12, and folate. They wonder if such a therapy regimen would also reduce the impact of Alzheimer's disease (AD) and slow the cognitive decline.

To find out, the National Institute on Aging is doing a study called Vitamins to Slow Alzheimer's, or VITAL. Sixty percent of the subjects will receive high doses of the three vitamins (5mg. of folate, 25 mg. of vitamin B6, and 1 mg. of vitamin B12) and 40 percent will receive an identical looking placebo. The study will last eighteen months, and participants will be examined for their performance on a test that evaluates cognitive functions, such as memory, attention, reasoning, and language.

DO FOODS PLAY A ROLE?

Nutrition research in recent decades has found a major link between the foods we eat and the state of our health. Not surprisingly then, some scientists are examining whether certain ingredients in foods may help ward off Alzheimer's.

Spicing It Up

Fans of Indian cuisine are probably familiar with curry, the yellowish powder that gives Indian food its hue and flavor. Curry comes from turmeric, which is the dried root of the plant Curcuma longa. Its yellow color comes from a plant ingredient called curcumin, a substance that has anti-inflammatory and antioxidative properties, which has been found to lower cholesterol. Some studies have shown it may help prevent certain cancers, too.

Animal studies now suggest that curcumin may be able to interfere with the brain damage involved in Alzheimer's as well. In laboratory studies and research on transgenic mice—mice that have been injected with mutated genes for Alzheimer's—scientists found that curcumin blocked the formation of beta amyloid oligomers and fibrils. Curcumin was also able bind to the small amounts of beta amyloid and block the formation of the destructive plaques typical of Alzheimer's.

The research was so intriguing that the National Institute on Aging has launched a small clinical trial to study the effectiveness and safety of curcumin in patients with mild to moderate Alzheimer's.

Healthy Fish Oils

For years, nutritionists have touted the perks of eating fish: It has less fat than meat and poultry; it can help lower cholesterol; and it may help keep cardiovascular disease at bay. But new research is suggesting that ingredients in fish such as salmon, mackerel, and herring may also protect against Alzheimer's disease.

Of particular interest are the omega-3 fatty acids, especially docosahexaenoic acid (DHA). Recent research on mice has found that a diet rich in omega-3s may guard against the memory loss involved in Alzheimer's, even when the disease is already evident in the brain. Researchers compared mice fed diets rich in DHA with those fed a diet low in DHA and those who received ordinary food. Results showed that mice fed diets rich in DHA had the lowest levels of beta amyloid.

To study the effects of fish oil in humans, the National Institute on Aging and the National Center for Complementary and Alternative Medicine are in the midst of a clinical trial evaluating the impact of fish oil on cognitive performance in patients with mild Alzheimer's.

CAN STATINS SLOW AD?

People who have high cholesterol are often given medications known as statins, a class of drugs chemically known as 3-hydroxy-3-methylglutaryl coenzyme A (HMG CoA) reductase inhibitors. These drugs reduce levels of low-density lipoprotein (LDL) cholesterol (which is the kind most strongly linked to coronary artery disease and stroke) by inhibiting a liver enzyme needed for the production of cholesterol. Drugs in this category include atorvastatin (Lipitor), fluvastatin (Lescol), lovastatin (Mevacor), pravastatin (Pravachol), and simvastatin (Zocor).

In recent years, scientists have begun to uncover a possible link between statins and Alzheimer's disease. Epidemiological studies found that taking statins, especially simvastatin, was associated with a decreased incidence of Alzheimer's. Prior studies had suggested that people with cardiovascular risk factors also seemed to be at greater risk for Alzheimer's. Other studies have shown that the apolipoprotein E (ApoE) gene that carries cholesterol through the body promotes the aggregation of beta-amyloid fragments into the amyloid plaques found in Alzheimer's. Experts speculate that statins may not only have a preventive effect on the disease, but also may help slow the progression of AD in patients who are already diagnosed.

Establishing the effectiveness of statins in combating Alzheimer's will require more research, including the drug's effects in people with normal cholesterol levels. At press time, the National Institute on Aging was recruiting patients for a multicenter trial of simvastatin. This is part of a study known as CLASP, or the Cholesterol Lowering Agent to Slow Progression (CLASP) of Alzheimer's Disease. The study will examine the effect of the drug in 400 patients with mild to moderate Alzheimer's.

WILL WE EVER SEE A VACCINE?

Dreams of a vaccine to protect against Alzheimer's have not completely vanished with the discontinuation of AN-1792, a vaccine under investigation by Elan Pharmaceutical. Early on, studies showed that the vaccine prevented the formation of plaques in the brains of young mice genetically engineered to produce amyloid and reduced the formation of plaque in older mice. In humans, the vaccine showed that some patients developed amyloid antibodies. The studies then went into a phase IIA trial that involved about 360 subjects with mild to moderate Alzheimer's.

Unfortunately, the vaccine trials were discontinued after four participants developed inflammation of the brain and spinal cord. Less then two months later, eleven subjects developed the same symptoms, and the trial came to an end.

Many scientists say the quest for an eventual vaccine is far from over. Some researchers are exploring ways to refine the AN-1792 vaccine, possibly by targeting a portion of beta amyloid rather than an entire fragment, which experts theorize might have caused the inflammation. Other researchers are looking for ways to interfere with the development of beta amyloid by stimulating the patient's immune system to identify and eliminate the destructive plaques, which is known as active immunization. Still others are exploring passive immunization—the administering of routine injections—as a way to prevent Alzheimer's.

Recently, scientists at the Johnnie B. Byrd Alzheimer's Center and Research Institute in Tampa, Florida, reported some promising results with a vaccine tested in transgenic mice. The mice were given routine beta amyloid immunization throughout most of their adult lives and then tested at two intervals: as adults and in old age. Results showed that the immunotherapy delivered partial, or even complete protection, against cognitive decline at both test points. The tests measured several different cognitive abilities including memory, working memory and recognition.

CAN ALZHEIMER'S BE PREVENTED?

Research is starting to show that Alzheimer's may be prevented with the right lifestyle choices. The good news is, the same strategies that keep diabetes, cardiovascular disease, and certain cancers at bay may also play a role in reducing your risk for Alzheimer's.

To encourage preventive lifestyle habits, the Alzheimer's Association launched the Maintain Your Brain campaign. Here are some strategies they suggest:

- *Keep your brain active every day.* Whether it's reading a good book, doing a crossword puzzle, or playing a game, mentally stimulating activities can keep your brain healthy.
- *Stay socially engaged.* You may want to continue working a little longer or engage in volunteer activities. Consider joining social groups that involve mentally and physically stimulating activities. Travel is another way to stay socially active.
- *Remain physically active.* Regular exercise helps maintain good flow to the brain. That doesn't mean you need to train for a marathon or commit to a strenuous workout every day. All you need is some aerobic exercise to improve oxygen flow to the brain, which can reduce brain cell loss. Taking a walk, bicycling, or gardening for about thirty minutes a day is all it takes to get the body moving and heart pumping. Taking a new route every few days and walking with a friend adds mental activity and social engagement to your workout.
- *Eat a brain-healthy diet.* Concentrate on eating less fat and cholesterol. Control portion sizes and calories, so that you manage a healthy body weight. Studies show that high cholesterol, high blood pressure, and obesity in middle age are all risk factors for Alzheimer's. Focus on eating more richly colored fruits and vegetables such as kale, spinach, broccoli, beets, red bell peppers, blueberries, blackberries, strawberries, raspberries, plums, oranges, red grapes, a~ cherries. Add cold water fish, which contain h

omega-3 fatty acids, and nuts, which contain healthy amounts of the antioxidant vitamin E.

CLINICAL TRIALS: SHOULD YOU ASSIST IN RESEARCH?

Advances in the treatment of Alzheimer's could not be achieved without the help of investigators. But the research wouldn't be possible without the participation of important people: the patients.

Before any medical treatment can be approved by the U.S. Food and Drug Administration, it requires several research studies to prove that the treatment is safe and effective. That's where clinical trials come in. Clinical trials, also called clinical studies, are carefully conducted research studies using human volunteers to answer specific questions about a treatment for a condition. The treatment might be a new vaccine, drug, medical device, or procedure. The trials are done after research in laboratories shows promising results in animals. The goal is then to find out how the new therapy or procedure will work in people, and to determine its risks and its effectiveness. Clinical trials also look at methods of prevention, diagnosis, screening, and ways to improve quality of life.

Several different kinds of organizations are involved in clinical trials, including doctors, medical institutions, pharmaceutical companies, foundations, and government agencies. The trials are conducted in various settings, ranging from a small doctor's office to a large university setting or hospital. All clinical trials are governed by an Institutional Review Board made up of an independent committee of physicians, community advocates, and others that oversees the ethics of the research, ensures that the rights of the participants are protected, and reviews the research on a periodic basis.

As a person with Alzheimer's, you might consider participating in a clinical trial of a treatment or procedure for the disease. By doing so, you might gain access to a medication that is not widely available. You may also enjoy medical care at leading health care facilities. Some people may feel they've exhausted all other options. For others, the altruism of contributing to science and medicine may be enough to convince them to join a clinical trial.

Before you can participate however, you have to make sure you qualify for the trial. Some people may be excluded because of age, gender, the stage of the disease, and other medical conditions. Some trials want candidates who have a certain condition. After meeting with the doctors and nurses involved in the trial, you will need to sign an informed consent document that says you understand the risks and benefits of participating.

Being part of a clinical trial does involve risks. Some participants might be given a placebo, or inactive treatment, which is used to gauge the treatment's effectiveness. If you do receive the treatment, you may experience unpleasant, even life-threatening side effects. You will also have to endure more frequent visits to the testing site, treatments, and hospital stays than normal. And for all the time and energy you invest, you may also find that the treatment has no beneficial effect on your condition.

To Help You Decide

According to clinicaltrials.gov, a Web site of the National Institutes of Health, there are several things you should know before you decide to participate in a clinical trial:

- What is the purpose of the study?
- Who is going to be in the study?
- Why do researchers believe the new treatment being tested may be effective? Has it been tested before?
- What kinds of tests and treatments are involved?
- How do the possible risks, side effects, and benefits in the study compare with the medications I'm currently taking for the disease?

- How might this trial affect my life?
- How long will the trial last?
- Will hospitalization be required?
- Who will pay for the treatment?
- Will I be reimbursed for other expenses?
- What type of long-term follow-up care is part of the study?
- How will I know if the treatment is working?
- Will I see the results of the trial?
- Who will be in charge of my care?

Before you make any final decision, talk to your physician, family members, and friends. Balance the positives with the negatives and gather information about specific trials. If you think you'd like to participate, check out www.clinicaltrials.gov, a Web site that has information about more than 8,000 clinical trials being conducted primarily in the U.S. and Canada, but also in some foreign sites. You might also contact doctors, hospitals, or health care organizations for information.

A FINAL NOTE

It's hard to predict when any of these research efforts will become a part of our medical care for Alzheimer's—or whether some ever will. But scientists are forging ahead with efforts to understand this disease that just a century ago didn't even have a name. The intensity of these efforts suggests that there is hope that one day we will gain control over this illness.

CHAPTER TWELVE ✌

Profiles

MARY LOCKHART

My name is Mary. I live in Oklahoma City, Oklahoma, with my husband of forty years. We have two sons and six grandchildren. Before I was diagnosed with Alzheimer's, I ran a licensed daycare center for infants. I had my business for fifteen years. I was really good at it too.

Then I noticed I wasn't able to remember when the babies had their bowel movements and other things that I never had problems remembering before. I was having problems with my speech and coming up with the right words. I was experiencing severe headaches with a sort of burning sensation inside my head. I would get lost going to the doctor's office. Inside a bathroom, I couldn't remember which door to go out of and sometimes, I couldn't figure out how to open the door to get out of the bathroom. If I went to the mall with someone and that person got out of my sight, it would scare me so bad I wanted to cry. My husband tried to get me to use the computer but I just couldn't follow what he was telling me. I used to type sixty-five words per minute. But then I couldn't even remember where the keys were.

At the age of 55, I decided to tell my doctor about my problems. Right away he sent me for an MRI. The MRI showed a large amount of shrinkage. He then referred me to a neurologist, who sent me for two days of testing. I got hit with my diagnosis of dementia of the Alzheimer's type. My husband and I were both in shock.

The doctor said I should give up my job. That was so hard for me to do because every morning I looked forward to those smiling babies. I went to see a social worker who was great in helping me work through everything. I still call her if I ever need her, and she is always there for me. And if she doesn't hear from me she will call and check on me.

Three years ago, I started taking Aricept, and I can't believe the change it made in my thinking ability. I am now able to use the computer and type. I have my own Web page, a daily journal, photos, and links to other patient's Web sites that was made for me by my husband. My husband is real supportive of me and when I complain, he always tells me we are in this together.

To fill the void of not having the babies to care for, I now have three little dogs. I also have an aquarium and enjoy feeding and watching the birds and squirrels. I read everything I can about the disease.

This is a very lonely disease. I don't want anyone to feel as lonely as I did when I received my life sentence. At the time I thought I was the only person in my fifties that had Alzheimer's, but now I know there are many of us. Helping others not to be so frightened when they get a diagnosis of Alzheimer's or other dementia is what I want to do.

It has always helped me to help others. I have always been a caregiver, being the oldest of seven children, and I need to feel useful. That's why in 2000 I co-founded Dementia Advocacy Support Network International, or DASNI. DASNI is a not-for-profit corporation "established to promote respect and dignity for persons with dementia, provide a forum for the exchange of information, encourage support mechanisms such as local groups, counseling groups and Internet linkages, and advocate for services for people with dementia."

I host chats at the Web site at www.alzinfo.org/chatrooms. Yes, I am still hosting chats every day. People who come to chat are mostly people with dementia or Alzheimer's. They come from New Zealand, United Kingdom, Australia, Canada, Brazil, Scotland, and all over the United States. Sometimes we have caregivers join in also. On Monday night we had a special guest, David Shenk, who is the author of *The Forgetting*. Most of the time, we discuss what kind of day we are having. If we have started a new medication, we might share that. We also talk about our families, hobbies, weather, favorite foods, and so on. We laugh and cry together. I wish they could have had something out there like that for me when I was diagnosed. I was told I only had five years to live by my neurologist. That was quite scary for my husband and me. Without DASNI, I would be a very lonely person.

My days aren't bad for the most part, though I do get easily fatigued. I try not to dwell on having Alzheimer's. But I do think of it when I look on the counter and see my pills that my husband has put out for me to take. I do see them but then think I need to put something away, or that I will take them as soon as I've run to the bathroom, and next thing I know, that is the end of the good thought of taking the medication on the counter.

Yes, I still take Aricept and that is all I take for the dementia. I believe my condition has declined some. I can no longer drive, or hold down a job, and I don't do housekeeping like I used to. I do very little around the house. I am still able to do laundry but no longer know how to iron. I can cook with help. I have made out my living will and given my husband power of attorney. And I have told my family when I get to be a burden to put me in a home.

I like to tell people that if you are having a bad day wait till tomorrow and it will be better. Also I have a cross stitch of a print made for me by a dear friend and it says: "When God Closes a Door, He Opens a Window." I read that so often. When I got Alzheimer's and could no longer work, God closed a door, but He opened a window and gave me more special time with my family.

JEANNE L. LEE

Jeanne Lee likes to say that she's living with Alzheimer's, not dying of it. Since her diagnosis in 1995, she has written a book, started a group for people in the early stages of Alzheimer's, and become a lecturer on the topic internationally and throughout Hawaii, where she lives, and has even traveled to Barcelona representing the U.S. at an international AD conference.

But her early struggles with the disease were difficult, and it took several years for Jeanne to get a proper diagnosis. In the five years before she was diagnosed, Jeanne lived in a state of constant confusion. While driving, she was would get lost on familiar roads. In the middle of a sentence, she'd find herself at a loss for words. She once came out of a doctor's office to find she had left her car running with the keys inside and the doors locked. To make matters worse, her moods were erratic. She would cry one minute and laugh the next, with no apparent reason for the abrupt change in mood.

At her job as an assistant manager of a printing center, she had trouble remembering how to operate the various machines. She would make phone calls and forget whom she'd called. If someone put her on hold, she wouldn't remember who the person was when he got back on the line.

The thought that she might have Alzheimer's struck her as a possibility. After all, her mother had had Alzheimer's, and Jeanne had seen her mom transform from a sweet, kind, gentle woman to a raging tyrant who cut up photographs of people who infuriated her, accused her children of stealing, and swore with shocking vulgarity. She eventually became so combative that she was placed in a nursing home. There, her mother was a calmer, happier person. When she died surrounded by family and friends, her mother was tapping her fingers to her favorite music.

But at 50, Jeanne, and most of her doctors, thought she was too young to have Alzheimer's. They gave her numerous brain scans, X-rays, and blood tests, but couldn't pin down a diagnosis. One doctor simply prescribed pills to her for a year but saw her in person only twice. Another told her to go home because he couldn't help her while she was sobbing.

Jeanne became increasingly depressed, especially after she botched a major job at the print center and decided she had to quit. She was embarrassed by her failing communication skills and her inability to be organized, and she found little joy or pleasure in anything she did. She became a recluse. Eventually, Jeanne was in such despair that she attempted suicide and wound up in a psychiatric hospital, where she was diagnosed with schizophrenia and depression.

Finally in 1995, a psychiatrist confirmed Jeanne's suspicions. Jeanne had Alzheimer's. Oddly enough, Jeanne was elated to get the news. "I truly jumped for joy (when I found out that) this thing that was turning my world upside down had a name," she says. "No more mental institutions for schizophrenia or depression, no more suicide attempts, no more begging doctors to check me out. Now I could tell all the people I had been hiding from because of embarrassment that I was not crazy, that the problem had a name. It was dementia of the Alzheimer's type."

Getting a formal diagnosis relieved the stress of not knowing what was wrong with her. But Jeanne continued to live with the symptoms of the disease. She bounced checks. She put Spam in her boyfriend's underwear drawer. She left her house without her partial dentures, and applied her partials with toothpaste instead of fixative. Eventually, she had to give up driving, cooking, and paying bills.

But rather than dwell on what she had to sacrifice, Jeanne says she's found new meaning in her life by focusing on what she can do and has discovered new purpose as an educator on Alzheimer's. These days, she gives lectures about Alzheimer's to local hospitals, churches, rotary clubs, and professional organizations. She speaks about four times a month. She has written a book about her experiences called *Just Love Me: My Life Turned Upside Down by Alzheimer's* (Purdue University Press, 2003). She also started an early stage support group, which grew from three members to nine in one month. The group has since disbanded, but members still call Jeanne with questions.

She has also started a business called Alzheimer's Awareness and Prevention, which she says is "dedicated to research and education of what cannot be learned from books by integrating the knowledge of all involved to include those who have AD and other dementias." Adds Jeanne, "We are striving to prove that an AD diagnosis may be a setback but it's not the end of life's journey. There can still be joy in one's life after diagnosis."

Jeanne also joined Dementia Advocacy and Support Network International, became an active member and now serves on the Board of Directors. "Talking to someone with the same problems and others who were diagnosed young was a hold on life for me," she says.

Being diagnosed with Alzheimer's has had profound effects on other aspects of her life, too. She began following a more natural diet and taking supplements such as gingko biloba for Alzheimer's and St. John's wort for depression, a combination of vitamins E and C, and vitamin B12. She started eating more fruits and vegetables and took up exercise.

After she regained some of her cognitive function, she also began reading more, not just books about Alzheimer's, but others about diverse topics, especially travel. She says she thought that the only way to prevent the knowledge she had from disappearing was to keep the brain going at full speed and working as long as possible. However, she is no longer able to read the newspaper or phone books. And when she does read books, she cannot recall what they are about. If she stops, she must start all over again in order to remember information from earlier chapters.

Jeanne has done a great deal of reading about Alzheimer's and is especially excited by the prospect that Alzheimer's may someday be prevented—she has five children and thirteen grandchildren. She spouts off information about healthy habits that can prevent or delay Alzheimer's: Watching TV takes less brain power than sleeping. Couch potatoes are more likely to have AD than people who are physically fit. Crossword puzzles are one of the great helps for the brain.

"My lectures are a huge part of slowing my own downhill slide," Jeanne says. "But anything one can do to remain in great health and avoid heart attacks is also good for preventing AD. That means keeping one's blood sugar, cholesterol, and body weight under control."

Jeanne also tries to educate family members, caregivers, and the general public on how to treat people who have Alzheimer's or dementia. "We're not here to convince you we have a dementia," she says. "Never say that you do something all the time when you really do it just a few times a year—we do it five to ten times an hour. Do not teach someone with dementia as if she is below you. Do not scold us if the things we do are wrong. Offer help but do not take over, as we are losing independence by the day."

Jeanne has a message for doctors too. "The medical field is our first hope for help," she says. "Do not cast us off without testing us with at least a Mini-Mental State Exam. You can't just label it depression without proper testing. An accurate diagnosis in the earliest stages of the disease is critical."

JUDY AND BUDDY

For years, Buddy and Judy Broadwater had looked forward to retirement. They owned property in the Smoky Mountains and were planning to build a chalet there. After years of hard work—he in law enforcement and she as a nurse—they planned to spend their retirement days alternating between the mountains and the beach.

Buddy, now 64, retired from his job as a United States postal inspector in 1990. Though he never became a lawyer, he did have a law degree, and at the age of 28, was the youngest police chief in the state of Alabama. In retirement, he was planning to work part-time as a consultant, doing background checks for various agencies such as the FBI.

But the joy of early retirement didn't last. Soon after, Buddy's health began to deteriorate. He suffered frequent headaches, and became nervous and anxious, something that was never part of his calm personality. Judy noticed a loss of enthusiasm and a flatness in his energy. "His highs were never quite as high, and his lows were never super low," Judy says. "And he used to be a man who did everything with gusto. A friend of mind even said, 'Where did Buddy's personality go?' At the time, it hurt my feelings, but I think it's because she was right."

Buddy was also experiencing memory lapses. "I would go into a room, say hello, and they'd say their name," he recalls. "Then I'd leave and forget their name."

At one point, Judy mistook his memory lapses as an insult after he repeatedly forgot their plans for weekend getaways. "I asked him one night, 'Does what I say not interest you, or is it that it's just not important enough for you to retain it?'" she says. To this day, she says she has regretted those words.

Buddy began going to doctors, who told him he was suffering panic attacks and anxiety. Judy began to suspect that her husband had Alzheimer's. But a PET scan by a neurologist and several visits to a psychiatrist assured her that he did not. In 1998, still looking for answers, the couple drove to a Mayo Clinic in Jacksonville, Florida, ninety-two miles away.

At Mayo, Buddy underwent four hours of testing. Under questioning, Buddy couldn't remember the date or the name of our nation's president. When asked to name the president who served before Clinton, he answered Roosevelt. He also had no memory of the couple's wedding anniversary—which happened to be that day—or the number of kids they had, for instance.

The doctors diagnosed Buddy with Alzheimer's. Because he was only 58 at the time, he was told he had early onset AD. One of the first issues the doctors discussed was driving. "When they told us it was Alzheimer's, they said he had to seriously consider giving up driving," Judy says. "And here he had just driven us down the highway to Mayo with me napping beside him."

After the diagnosis, the couple went out for lunch and tried to eat. "Buddy just held his head down and said, 'I am so sorry that this is what I'm going to put you through,'" Judy recalls. That night, in her first journal entry, Judy wrote, "Happy anniversary, darling. We have Alzheimer's."

Buddy quit working three days later, but the couple didn't discuss the matter of Buddy's driving for three weeks. Finally, Judy announced one night that they had to resolve the driving question the next day. "That night, the car keys were on my pillow," she says. "Of course I didn't sleep that night. I just cried and cried. But Buddy just said, 'If that's what I have to do then that's what I just have to do.'"

Buddy was left home alone while Judy continued working, She began returning home to some strange surprises. One day, Buddy used super glue to attach a rock emblazoned with the word 'Welcome' to the wall. Another time, she came home to find a chair had been freshly spray painted. He also started promising a lot of money to telemarketers on the telephone until Judy got caller I.D. and taught him to screen the phone calls.

Attempts to slow the disease with medications such as Aricept and Namenda didn't work, and Judy was becoming increasingly worried about leaving Buddy home alone. But she was reluctant to give up her job as a nurse for an insurance company, which was now the couple's sole source of income. Her work entailed a great deal of travel, so Buddy began going with her and staying in the hotels.

On one particular trip, the couple brought their granddaughter too, and Judy took the little girl to see a movie. While turning into the hotel parking lot, her cell phone rang. It was the local police. Buddy had reported her missing. "I knew that Buddy would never have done that before," Judy says. "But I had begged God to give me a sign when it was time for me to quit. And I knew that that was my sign." Judy quit that day in June 2002 and has since spent virtually every moment of her life with Buddy.

A great deal has changed over the years. Instead of watching educational television and news programs as he used to do, Buddy became more interested in half-hour sitcoms. He stopped reading in bed at night and began to favor word searches instead of the crossword puzzles he used to do. Once an avid golfer, he cut back from eighteen holes to nine. And he no longer does paintings—he did landscapes and still lifes—as frequently as he once did.

Relationships with friends and family changed, too. Though they remain close to their son and his family, their daughter has kept her distance as has Buddy's sister, whom Judy suspects may also be developing Alzheimer's, but who denies that anything is wrong. Old friends who Judy thought would stick around have since disappeared as Alzheimer's has crept into their lives. "I was profoundly disappointed," Judy says. "These were some very educated people who have just slowly backed out of our lives."

Making new friends, she says, is impossible unless the new acquaintances understand Alzheimer's or are experiencing it right now. One of her best friends now is a woman who is caregiving for her husband. The two women talk on the phone almost every night.

Finding time away from Buddy is difficult. Judy says they can't afford the $14 an hour she'd need to pay an in-home aide. The brief breaks she does get come from an adult day care program run by the local Council on Aging, where Buddy goes twice a week for four hours at a time.

"He thinks he's volunteering there," she says. "They play bingo and do art projects. And he does push an old lady around in a wheelchair or directs people to the rest rooms. But somewhere deep down, I think he knows the truth because he always tells me, 'You go and do something for yourself.'" In those times, Judy runs errands, does her grocery shopping and occasionally gets a haircut.

These days, Buddy says he can tell he's getting worse. Simply mustering the energy to start a painting for a former golf buddy feels impossible. "I used to love to paint, and I've got a picture here that I'd like to paint, but I just can't push myself to do it," he says. "It tires me out just knowing that it would tire me out. So I have everything set aside, and the day will come when I will finish it."

Judy fears that Buddy is moving from the early stages of the disease into the more advanced stages. His food preferences are becoming more child-like, and his latest favorite is peanut butter and jelly sandwiches, which are the only thing he can still prepare, albeit sloppily. Recently, he declared that he is no longer eating broccoli or lima beans. If there's something sweet on his plate, he always eats that first.

The other day, Judy took Buddy to the supermarket, where he was putting all kinds of sugary cereals into the shopping cart and begging for lemon drops. "It's just so un-Buddy like," she says. "I have a real hard time accepting un-Buddy. He's always been my rock."

His grooming habits are slipping, too. During his morning routine, he frequently forgets to put on his deodorant and needs a reminder to brush his teeth. His shaving is uneven and sloppy, and Judy usually needs to freshen it up afterward with an electric razor. To ensure he wears the right clothes for the climate, Judy lays out his outfits every morning.

With every lost skill, Judy says she goes through a mourning period that parallel the stages of grief. At first she denies that anything is changing, then she gets angry, frustrated, and sad. Finally, she finally learns to accept that her husband has slipped yet again.

Each day, Buddy follows a regular routine that starts off with feeding squirrels at a nearby McDonald's. During the day, he watches TV, but has trouble following the story lines. At every commercial break, he gets up and walks away, thinking the show is over until Judy reminds him that there's still more to come. Throughout the day, Buddy repeats himself over and over again, and by the end of each afternoon, Judy says she is thoroughly exhausted.

With all her experience as a caregiver, Judy occasionally leaves Buddy at a friend's house to teach a class on caregiving strategies for the local Alzheimer's Association chapter. Don't rush the patients. Give them one instruction at a time. Do things that still bring them joy. Help them get their exercise and eat well. Keep a journal for yourself. "I'm trying to teach them coping skills," Judy says. "I'm also teaching them that among the tears, there's still a lot of laughter. If you can't laugh, then the party is over."

In her own life, Judy, who is 62, strives to maintain a sense of humor. Asked if Buddy helps around the house for instance, she quips, "It depends on how aggravated I want to be. He still does the garbage, but sometimes, he'll just bag it and leave it sitting there, and I have to remind him to finish the job."

Once, she recalls with a laugh, her son took Buddy golfing. Buddy and her son teamed up with two other men on the golf course, and in the middle of the game, Buddy started hitting the other players' balls. And she chuckles when she sees Buddy outside competing with his six-year old grandson to see who can kick a soccer ball farther. "You've got your grandchildren going forward and your husband going backward," Judy says.

The future used to be a source of tremendous concern for Judy. Early on, the couple made out a will, appointed Judy durable power of attorney, took Buddy's name off all the checking accounts, and arranged to have all checks sent to Judy. "I used to try and plan for the future, but now I just don't worry about it," she says. "If he holds, I can hold."

As for Buddy, he says he doesn't give any thought to the future any more. "I just want life to be as simple as it can be, and to take it day by day," he says. And he certainly doesn't live in the past. "The things I've forgotten I wouldn't want to even try to remember because it's too frustrating," he says.

Living in the present is one of the blessings Judy has learned from her husband's experience with Alzheimer's. Even his blood pressure has dipped since he's let go of the many things that used to stress him out. At the beach, he admires the blue skies and gazes at every passing bird. He turns over seashells and studies the patterns. "He is so much more in touch with life than I am," she says. "He is stopping and smelling the roses. It makes me stop and say, 'Okay, he's right. This is not a race. This is a walk.'"

CHIP GERBER: A JOURNAL

I was born in Dover, Ohio, many years ago. Back in 1997, at the age of 51, I was diagnosed with Early-Onset Alzheimer's Disease. I was a few years from retirement, although I tended not to think about it. I enjoyed what I did for a living. I had been a social worker for over twenty-five years, and also served as youth director and pastor in different churches.

In my last job, I was a court-appointed guardian for senior citizens. I assessed the cases and would serve my agency in court as a witness to the situation. I was well known in my community and in the probate court system.

Then my memory began to complicate my job. I could no longer follow notes or even keep up with the paper work. I could no longer concentrate or remember details. I was getting behind. I began to panic, to have anxiety attacks, to lose control. I became clinically depressed. What was happening to me? What did I have? What was causing my memory loss and making me unable to carry out my assignments?

After being hospitalized on several occasions and many visits with my doctor, the mystery was given a name. I was told I had the beginning of Alzheimer's disease and put shortly thereafter on Aricept. I could only work part time.

A year and a half ago, I went to Mayo Clinic for complete testing by the head of the neurology department. The doctor diagnosed me with Lewy body dementia, then recently changed it to Alzheimer's disease with Lewy body components. He increased my dosage of Aricept.

Arrangements have been made for my wife to have power of attorney, and a living will has been arranged. We have talked to an attorney and tried to make all the arrangements we could while I can still contribute to the decision-making.

I keep active with simple chores, family, and friends. Church and support groups also assist me along with the computer and reading. I'm trying to stretch my mind as much as possible and keep as active as my energy allows.

I've found that having a great caregiver like my wife Sharon, being flexible, laughing as much as possible, and getting lots of rest in between keeps me going. I am slowing down considerably, but am far from dead. I journal, not as much as I once did, but still enough to keep my mind active and others encouraged, I hope.

Fear? No. By dealing with the issues early, I have found I do not fear the disease. I do get frustrated and angry during moments. I fight depression but am usually able to keep positive. I know the final stages of this disease, but refuse to dwell there. I still have living to do. Who knows where this adventurous journey will take me yet?

Chip has given us permission to reprint portions of his journal here. It is still available on-line at http://www.zarcrom.com/users/ alzheimers/chip.html.

February 4th, 2001

When I was a child, my Mom always emphasized the importance of wearing clean underwear when I left the house. If anything happened to me before I returned, she wanted to make sure I had clean underwear on.

These days before I leave my home I think of other things. Have I turned off the lights and all the burners? Do I have my keys, my billfold, my money, handkerchief, and comb? Do I have important addresses and phone numbers, glasses, and spare keys? I'm tired before I leave. It's quite a process. And then, yes, I want to have on clean underwear too. Some advice tends to stick. It's just the everyday things that leave.

February 8th, 2001

I was just thinking, who's counting anyway? I forgot to change my socks again. I forgot to take my medication. I forgot what you just said. I slept in an extra hour this morning. Okay? I admit that I did these things.

They happened. I forgot to say thank you when I should have yesterday and recently I forgot to take a bath. Now, I wouldn't want to forget my bath very often, but for a day, who's counting?

Yes, I forget. No new news here. Was it Alzheimer's that caused the slip? Perhaps it was because I was under stress or because I'm getting a bit older. Does one and one have to always equal two? Must I continually be reminded that I have a type of dementia? There are moments when I want to forget that I have this disease. I might be a tad bit frustrated at the moment. I don't want to be reminded that I am ill. I realize that I am sick and that as a result, some negative things are going to happen in my life, but I refuse to live there, to dwell on it. I choose to go on living, and go on living I will. For me that means at times I must leave my diagnosis in the background and press on with life.

February 9th, 2001

I thought I would give you an update on my mother, Mary, who is soon to be 87. About three months ago she was placed in an assisted living facility for those with impaired memory. Mom had many bruises from falling when she was cared for by family. My sister, Anna, cared for my mother for many years and did the best she could possibly do for her. There came a time and place when my mom had to take the next step and move to get the care that she required.

I had mixed feelings about the move, but wanted the best for my mother. The home had a good reputation and seemed to be right for her. I must say after watching carefully for three months that it was the right thing to do. No matter how unpleasant it is for my mother or members of the family, it was the right thing to do and the right time to do it.

Three months later I am content with the family decision. Mom is beginning to walk with the help of a walker again, which she had not been able to do for some time. She appears to be well cared for and I can be with her any time that I choose.

Mom, having Alzheimer's disease for many years now, cannot understand why she is living there and asks about returning home. These are difficult moments because although going home is what I would want for her, it cannot be. Her needs are best cared for at this location. Although I will probably always feel bad about her being there, I am glad there is such a place and am grateful for the TLC that is given to my mom. At some point, I too may need this care myself.

February 10th, 2001

It was a rainy day and I would've just as soon stayed inside the house, but I ventured out to attend a class with some friends. We were driving along when all of a sudden we saw a rainbow. I could see both ends of it, and it was beautiful. It made me glad that I ventured out. It made me glad to be alive. To me a rainbow is not only something of beauty, but it is a reminder for me. It reminds me that as I journey onward that someone is holding my hand and is there for me. It's a reminder to me that I don't have to live in fear and that life is not over for me. I can face an uncertain tomorrow because He cares.

February 12th, 2001

I was thinking about my memory and what I recall. For example, I recall where I was and who I was with yesterday. Supper is still very vivid. But the rest of the day is gone. The day before is fading fast. It was Sunday, but my recollection is very fuzzy of what I did. I remember going to church, but that is something we do each week. The occurrences from the day before are gone. And before that is lost...I can still recall bits of events usually, but the details disappear quickly. For me this is a huge loss. At one time I was very good with details.

An old saying is, "Don't cry over spilled milk." I'm not exactly crying or even complaining, I'm just sharing and somehow that is different and very soothing for me. I don't mind sharing. Crying and complaining I try not to do often. Only happens by accident.

February 13th, 2001

Former President Ronald Reagan had his ninetieth birthday recently. His wife, Nancy, was asked if the day would be special. She stated that it would just be another day. Made me think. We that have Alzheimer's Disease have those every day. Just another day. Life goes on, but not too eventful. Day after day, week after week. We may have a special occasion here and there but mostly it's just another day.

For me, this is why I must have the right attitude. It helps me to look for the simplicity of life, the uniqueness and the spiritual aspects of life. This somehow can add a little extra to just another day. I want more than just another day. I insist that there be meaning to my daily existence and you know what? I find it.

February 16th, 2001

I was thinking about masks today. We all wear them. Hide behind them. It's not easy to be open, to be honest with each other about things and issues that are close to us. It's so much easier to stay hidden, unexposed. This way we do not have to explain, we can stay uninvolved and take glances from a distance. Sort of like sitting in church....did I say that?

I do believe that some spend their entire lives in hiding. But who are we hiding from? I believe it is not just from others, but perhaps from ourselves also. By hiding from ourselves, our true feelings, we don't have to deal with them. We will never truly know ourselves, and others will never really know us unless we take off our masks.

When it comes to Alzheimer's Disease, we can spend the rest of our existence in denial, or we can come out and examine who we have become, where we are presently, and where we go from here.

To me, this is what chatting on my computer is about. This is what I want my early onset Alzheimer's Disease monthly meeting to be about. If I wanted a tea party I would stay at home and have one, but I don't. I want reality. I want to discuss the issues we all face moment by moment. There may be moments of silence, of crying, or even of laughing, but I want these moments to be worthwhile, to be real and honest. A time to think, to reflect, to feel, to share, and when I am uncomfortable or just desire it, a privilege to hide for a time. Please allow me to do this. Please help create a safe place for me that I might mourn, share, reshape, grow, develop, then dance and hopefully fly. I am counting on you.

February 17th, 2001

I was thinking about how fast life goes by. It seems to fly by. I think of those that are gone, a father, brother, grandparents on both sides of the family, my mother-in-law and father-in-law. Many friends through the years. It seems not long ago that they were here with me, a very important part of my life.

We occasionally drive into Amish country, which is not far from where we live. It's like walking into another time, another day, another life. I love it. It's like a breath of fresh air. I watch cars fly down the roads and pass the horse and buggies that appear to almost be standing still. Usually both make it. The old and the new. The slow and the fast. Side by side.

My existence has slowed down considerably. And I like it. The rat race I was in not long ago has changed to a snail's pace. At first I was in shock and deeply offended by the change. Change can be difficult and I was never one that enjoyed it very much. But now it's like a breath of fresh air to me. I can do this. Yes, life has changed, it has slowed down for me, but I'm adjusting, and liking it more every day. I think I can get used to the change.

February 19th, 2001

Thought I'd let you in on a secret. Sharon and I went shopping today. I bought a brand new suit. Dark charcoal. Nice, very nice. Haven't had a new suit in the longest time. Well, I have to look nice on my upcoming trip to Washington, D.C. Me, in Washington! Well, Sharon, too of course. We're like twins. Where I go, she goes, and vice versa. I don't mind a bit. I love the woman. Soulmates forever.

Anyway, I was invited by the Alzheimer's Association in Washington, D.C. to give a five minute testimony, along with some others, before the House Appropriations Committee, who is conducting a series of meetings they call "Public Witness Hearings." What an honor and a privilege! I couldn't say no. I talk in my sleep for longer than five minutes. I'll be prepared with notes and all. That should keep me from rambling. Oh, and I better take along a five minute timer with me. Ha. If I can share my life and ask that they open up their hearts and funds for Alzheimer's Disease research, it will all be worth it. Boy, I only hope it helps. Somehow I feel it will.

My speech might be something like this: "Mr. President, Mr. Vice-president, Congressmen, Representatives...I'm Chip Gerber from Canton, Ohio, just an ordinary guy who feels very privileged to be here today. I'm being asked to come because I am one of the four million Americans that has Alzheimer's Disease.

"In the prime of life, at age 51, I was diagnosed as having something that most Americans cringe at. Alzheimer's Disease, a thief that steals, destroys, and kills. The disease has no cure and will take my life in a matter of years. I have been robbed of the ability to think well, to remember, to judge. I can no longer drive or be employed at what I loved to do, social work. My energy is low from the battle I am in. And yet, I do not come to ask for your pity or sympathy. I do not come here to complain, but only to remind you that I am one of a multitude. I could be anyone, your mate, your child, your friend. The disease does not discriminate. It strikes young and old. More and more of us are younger. I am 55. Around ten percent of the Alzheimer's Disease populations are below the age of 60. Our numbers are getting larger and will continue to increase as the years go by unless a cure is found.

"I have a dream. It is the same as the Alzheimer's Association. This dream is that within this generation there will be a cure for this deadly disease. I am one of three generations in my family now to have Alzheimer's Disease. My grandmother had it, my mother has it, and now I have it. If we act now, perhaps we can save my children and grandchildren from experiencing this awful fate, along with multitudes of others. Who among us will get it next?

"Last year a start was made. It was appreciated. The government did see fit to give some funds for Alzheimer's Disease research. This year we are requesting more. The goal of the Association is to receive one billion dollars over a two-year period. The lives that you save will be worth the effort and the dollars. It will be used well. The research that this will pay for may well bring about the cure that will end this terrible, deadly disease.

"I ask that you consider the effects of Alzheimer's Disease for which there is no cure. I'm told that an expert multi-professional

team is in place waiting for your approval of funds that can bring
about the cure that we so desire. With all respect, we are counting
on you to make the difference. Thank you for allowing me to
share from my heart."

Oh my, I did it! Did I go over my minutes? I know the speech
must be polished a bit, but that might be how it goes. I'll let you
know later. Wish me well. Your prayers will help too.

February 21st, 2001

Some time ago, I was attending a lecture at a local nursing home.
I continue to keep my social worker's license and must obtain
thirty credits of continuing education every two years to keep it
active. The social worker at the home offered to give us a tour of
a new Alzheimer's Unit they had just opened recently. I decided on
the spur of the moment that I would take this tour.

Now as a social worker, I worked with individuals who had
Alzheimer's Disease and had been placed in nursing homes. I have
had many classes in the past on Alzheimer's Disease and know how
to work with the client as well as the family. This was the first time
since my diagnosis that I've been back to an Alzheimer's unit in a
nursing home. I hadn't really thought about this before my tour.

The new unit was great. Very homey, cheerful, colorful with
many activities for those living there. I was impressed with the unit
and kidded later that I might want to be placed there when the
time comes.

When the time comes. What a thought. That is a place
where I don't allow my mind to wander often. But for this one
occasion I thought it wouldn't hurt me and it didn't. I was
pleased to see how active those in the unit were and what good
care they seemed to receive. I was impressed with the cheerful-
ness and openness of the unit and the staff. I'm very content to
stay in the earlier stages of my disease and am in no hurry to get

to the later stages, but when the times comes, and my wife can no longer care for me in the home, I want her to take me to a place such as this where I can live out my days. I do not want her to feel sorry or guilty in any manner. I want my wife to think of her own well-being and do what needs to be done. Before the time comes, I have made my decision to do what is best for my wife and my family, and really, the best for me. I know that this decision will not be easy.

February 22nd, 2001

Yesterday, early in the morning, I was attending the last class I need to meet the requirements to keep my social worker's license for two years.

The class was very interesting, but oh, so close to home. But still, it was informative and interesting and I needed that last 1½ credits.

It was a relief to get the last class completed. Each year it becomes more difficult to do. The desire is there, but the energy level is not. I've had the license for so many years that it is difficult for me to let it go. I've had the license ever since licensing began in our state.

I don't know how many more years I will struggle to keep it. Time can only tell. I do know that it is still meaningful to me and that it is a challenge. Perhaps soon it will become too much of a challenge. The material covered in the class is more difficult to comprehend and it is not easy to sit for the period I must sit. And I do not remember much of the presentations that I hear.

February 24th, 2001

Last night Mom asked me a question that about broke my heart. She asked, "You're not just trying to get rid of me, are you?" Mom is struggling with being in an assisted living facility. She is unable to understand. What she does understand is that she is no longer at home. I do my best to explain, knowing that whatever I say is not sufficient and will not be remembered long. But I try.

Why is she there? A good question. I would ask the same question if I were in her situation. We all want to be home. There's no place like home. Mom has spent eighty-six years of her life at home with family. Now she is in an unfamiliar setting with faces that she does not recognize. The family no longer had an option.

It's so easy to get upset with Mom's repetitious questions and to become flippant with our answers, but she deserves more. So much more. She deserves patience, respect, and understanding. No, it is no longer home and she'll never be able to understand that, but in our hearts we know that this has become her new home and that all her needs are being met here. That has to satisfy us at this time, although somehow, it is a hollow feeling. It still pulls at my heart strings. I can understand. It will never be home for her.

March 3rd, 2001

I was looking at some of my typing. Sometimes I murder the words. You should see my daily journal entry before Sharon proofreads and corrects it. Then again, maybe you shouldn't. My fingers just don't type what I want them to. There are times that I don't say what I want to either. At times I think I say one thing but I really said another thing, and there are occasions when I don't complete my thought or leave out something important.

How can I expect another individual to completely understand me? Well, I don't always, except for my wife, Sharon, who I expect to read between the lines. I expect her to be a mind reader. In fact she is usually pretty good at it too. To be all that I need her to be for me, I do appreciate this.

Caregivers will have stars in their crown someday for putting up with us. Sharon's crown will especially shine.

March 5th, 2001

It was a difficult feeling to describe. I was lost. I had gone to the restroom and was absent only a short time. Sharon and I were at a meeting together in an unfamiliar place. I had never been there before. It was a large building. Someone had pointed the way to the restroom and then left me. I felt sure I could find my way back. When I left the men's room I turned right. I went up the hall and found all doors were locked. There was no one available to ask for directions. I returned the way I thought that I had come and turned down another hallway. Still I found that I was in the wrong area.

I began feeling strange. I suddenly recalled being lost for a short time as a child. I was shopping with my mother who was giving more attention to the merchandise than she was to me. I was having a wonderful time. I was getting lost among the clothes, and soon I was really lost. The feelings of despair set in. And then I saw my mother, still shopping a distance from me. I remember running to her as fast as my legs would carry me, glad that I had found her. Oh what a relief it was.

Back to my recent journey. I hadn't given up and was still looking to find my way back to Sharon. Suddenly I saw a large opening. On the other side of it I could hear the sounds of many voices. As I got closer, I knew I was going in the right direction. Then I spotted some of the group that I had been sitting with earlier. They didn't seem to have missed me, but boy, I missed them. There was Sharon. What a relief it was to see her. I hadn't been gone long enough to be missed, so she hadn't come looking for me. The feelings of being lost soon left and were replaced by the excitement of being at the State Capital for the Memory Day Luncheon.

March 6th, 2001

The waitress said that it would be five dollars and some odd cents. I rooted through my billfold for the money. I also looked in my pocket for the needed change, but I had forgotten to bring any with me. I gave the waitress ten dollars and waited for change. It seemed like the longest wait. Then I began wondering, did I give her a ten or twenty dollar bill? I really couldn't recall. I was finally given my change. It was for ten dollars. But wait, I think I gave her twenty dollars. I guess I'll never know for sure. I must depend on the honesty of others in these situations. I have no other choice. I don't mind leaving a nice tip for the waitress, but I do need the money for bills.

When you can no longer remember, it sure can create a lot of problems. I try not to carry much money with me because I know that I will either have difficulty paying my bill, or I will question the change. My wife normally pays the bills for us. She writes all the checks. I reverse numbers and letters, and this can be dangerous when it comes to money matters.

The dilemmas that come with Alzheimer's are unending. The challenges are constant. It seems we are always relying on others for help. I don't think that I will ever be comfortable having to rely so much on others for help, but I am glad I can count on it when I need it.

March 7th, 2001

There are times when words just don't come out like I intend them to. The other day I had mashing instead of meshing. I was thanking rather than thinking. And then there are times that I refer to the stove rather than the refrigerator. Worse yet, there are times when nothing comes. I am interrupted in mid-sentence and the words are just not there. No wonder I get irritated! It makes me feel better when I hear comments from others, like "I understand." It also helps if someone asks me if this is what I meant to say. Most people are very caring and gracious.

My wife, Sharon, at times has to be a mind reader. She hears many times, "you know what I mean." Not a question, but a comment. Poor thing. And she usually does know what I'm trying to say. So many times she is able to fill in what I am unable to communicate. Sharon and I have been married for over twenty-five years. We seem to think a lot alike. At least, I'd like to think that we do.

March 12th, 2001

When it comes to doing a presentation, I set aside time to prepare. I've been going over my notes for the testimony in Washington, D.C. I do want to be prepared and ready for this event. I'm only allowed five minutes. I had Sharon time my presentation and it comes out to nine minutes. Now I tend to read slow and this just won't do. And then there is the very real possibility that I might lose my place. I am learning to place a finger on the line that I am on. And then I must remember to move my finger to the next line. Oh, what challenges I have. Little things can create big problems when we forget to do them. Things that those without the disease would never think about.

I hope to put some feeling, some life into my testimony. It's a message I care deeply about and I want it to come out that way. Not just read a presentation. I have a simple message: We are many and we need help and quickly.

March 13th, 2001

This is the day we depart for Washington, D.C. Sharon and I are prepared and excited about the journey. We are anxious for the challenge that lies ahead. We are traveling from the Akron-Canton Airport and we will change planes at Pittsburgh. From there we will go on to Washington, D.C. where we will be met by a staff person from the Washington Alzheimer's Association.

I believe in the team approach. No one person can get it all done. But together we can do it. Together we can make a difference.

My wife, Sharon, is very important in making my many plans happen. Without her help little would be accomplished. She gets a lot of the credit.

I have prepared and said my prayers, asking for the Lord's help and now I sit back and watch it happen. I am only one of the army that is assembled and ready to do battle, but as the old song says, "Little is much, when God is in it." There are many of us who have dementia who want our world to know about the disease, and we are not afraid to ask for help. I feel that as the days go by, more and more help will be on the way and that the outcome of our asking will be beyond our imaginations.

March 14th, 2001

We got up early to prepare for the day. We had a small breakfast at the hotel. I'm unable to eat much before a presentation. My stomach was churning slightly. We were then able to relax in the hotel lobby before we were met by a staff member from the Washington Alzheimer's Association. This office is part of the national headquarters and deals with public policy.

The testimony took place at the House of Representatives. The room was overflowing with advocates from varied backgrounds who were giving testimony, also requesting funding for their causes. A Mr. Nick met us and told us that I would be the eighth person to speak out of thirty people giving testimony.

The testimonies were interesting and really got my attention. The needs in that room were heart wrenching. Soon it was my turn. I tried to put out of my mind that the room was full of people and focus my attention on why I was there and who I was addressing. I had only five minutes to do this. What a challenge! First, I had to make sure I didn't lose my place on my notes so that I could include all my thoughts, but I also wanted to look into the eyes of those to whom I was speaking. Somehow I felt I was able to do this very thing. I felt they listened intently to what I had to say, which resulted in questions at the end of my testimony. The five minute alarm had gone off and I didn't even notice. I spoke for perhaps an additional minute or two to finish what I had begun. Many cameras were going off as I spoke, but I tried to center my attention not on them, but on the committee.

The time flew by so quickly. I have to admit I was a little nervous, but the longer I spoke, the more I became adjusted, realizing that I was on a mission, that I was given an opportunity to share what it is to experience Alzheimer's on a day-to-day basis, and to encourage my government to support us so that research can continue at an accelerated level to find a cure.

I felt good and the comments received from the Alzheimer's Association staff as well as others were positive. We then went on to celebrate what had just taken place.

March 18th, 2001

Sharon says I can't follow instructions. This is very true. Now there are reasons. I didn't hear you is one of them. Another is that I got mixed up. Or they were too confusing or too long. Perhaps I tried and it just didn't work. Or then there is the reason where I just didn't like the directions you gave me. Oh my... not me. Well, there are times....

I'm not trying to think of excuses. I know it probably looks that way. I'm just saying that many times there are reasons for us not following instructions. Have patience with us. It might take a little time. You might have to present the instructions at a different time or with other words to get our attention. Don't give up on us. In time, if we are able, we will follow the directions. Perhaps it would be best to make the directions into suggestions.

March 25th, 2001

I tend to forget, so before I forget what I learned or was told, I must write it down, if I can find my glasses, paper, and pen. Then after I write it down I must remember where I put it so that when I need it again, I know where to go to get what I wrote down. Then I must find my glasses and the paper where I wrote the message. I recently bought a nice, large spiral notebook to keep notes in. I was sure this was a good place to keep notes and things that I wanted to recall, but at the moment I have no idea where the notebook is.

All in a day I say. When I find it, I find it. I used to think everything must have a place, but I forget where that place is. I'm unable to learn a new place and have forgotten the old place. At times this becomes a real dilemma. A real problem. I refuse to think about this difficulty long because it can be upsetting to me and can lead to undesirable changes, like a headache.

I like to think of it this way. Each moment, each hour, and each day is an adventure. Step by step and day by day. This is how I must approach life. I cannot take myself or life too seriously. I must be able to see the funny side of life, so if you hear me laughing, laugh along with me. At times it's either laugh or cry and men aren't supposed to cry, are we?

I talk to myself more than I used to also. Sometimes it's just good self talk. At times I might even give a yell, when I'm alone, of course. I do have my pride. Well, then again, a lot of that has gone by the wayside too, but there is some that holds on. There are moments when I begin to feel sorry for myself, but then I begin thinking about all of those that are worse off than I am. And there are so many. I am blessed, and I count my blessings daily. This disease can sure help us see life as it really is.

April 4th, 2001

Sharon prepared chow mein noodles with chicken and vegetables for dinner yesterday. When we opened up the can of dried noodles, there were peanuts mixed up with them. Now, I've never seen them that way before, so I looked at the contents and peanuts were not listed. My mate asked if I put the peanuts in the dry noodles and I couldn't recall doing it. In fact, I was certain that I did not. My mate did not do it and no one else lives with us. Who is to blame? Well, don't look at me! I do some strange things sometimes, and don't recall doing it. But I really don't think I did that, did I? I've never done anything strange like that before, have I? No, not me. I wouldn't have, would I? I hear that we can do some pretty strange things, but I'm not ready for that. I'm not in that stage....I just don't do things like that...the time may come, but I will know when that time is....won't I?

It gets so confusing at times. I'm not as sure as I used to be, but I'm still pretty confident that I did not do it. It was not me, it was someone else....so there! Perhaps I should not be as certain as I once was. Maybe it's time to be more open to possibilities that it just might have happened.

I may have done it, or said it, but I probably didn't. Did I?

April 19th, 2001

I was with a room full of volunteers at a recognition luncheon earlier today, arranged by the Canton Alzheimer's Association. It was an exciting event.

Volunteers are ordinary people like you and me who care enough to give of their time and themselves to help others. I was blessed to be a part of that great company of people. We don't have to be touched by a disease to volunteer. But that should not keep us from volunteering either.

I love volunteering. The problem is that now that my disease has progressed and that I no longer drive, my wife, Sharon, is auto- matically volunteered when I volunteer. The other day I was at a meeting and I volunteered my time to shop for a gift for someone who had adopted a child. A lady near to me said loudly that by volunteering I meant that Sharon would do the shopping. Well, in a way that is correct, although I will be glad to go with her and help her with the gift purchase. Is this what the Bible meant when it said that two shall become one flesh? Well, I mean well anyhow.

I want to be busy helping others, and of course, my wife also enjoys doing the same. It's just that what I do almost always affects her as well.

Hey, two volunteers for the price of one!

April 21st, 2001

I hate it when people look right past me to the one next to me to ask a question about me. On occasion that happens. It's like I'm not really there, or I can't talk or respond myself. I'm sure they mean no harm, but it's just the idea. I can still talk. I can still think and have my own opinion and ideas. I have something to say and enjoy saying it. So when you see me, look into my eyes and ask me, talk to me, share with me as well as the person I might be with.

April 30th, 2001

I really enjoy journaling. I've been doing it now since July 18 of last year. I haven't missed many days. When I do miss a day I catch up, sending them on to our webmaster who does such a great job.

We have a counter on the website that I enjoy looking at. It shows me how many individuals have been on my site. The last I saw it had over 14,000 hits. To me that's very exciting. I journal because it is good for me. I also journal because I enjoy sharing and encouraging others. My wife, Sharon, has the difficult job of deciphering the journal entry that I do daily. Lord help her! She sure needs it to make sense out of the mess that I give her. But make sense out of it she does and she does a fine job, let me say. Thanks, Honey, for all the work you do to make it go for me.

There is a lot involved in journaling. Not only my time and energy, but that of two others besides myself. But it's worth every bit of it. I so enjoy the notes I get from around the globe. I've received notes from as far away as Canada, Australia, and Switzerland. The notes inspire me, make me laugh, and make me want to do more. Some are from those affected by the disease or other diseases, some from caregivers, some from family and friends. I recently received my first two notes from children. I was so impressed! Keep them coming folks. Sharon puts them in a scrapbook for me so that when I can no longer do what I do, I can enjoy the notes from you and hopefully recall better days and times. Memories are so important to me. And I sure have a lot of good ones. May we each spend the time we have left making good memories for us and those we love.

June 2, 2001

Oh, so close and yet just a bite away. I was hungry and had not had my lunch yet. I went to our cupboard, looked quickly, and pulled out what I thought was a can of tuna fish. Now I happen to like a tuna sandwich now and then, and it makes for a quick lunch. Noel, our cat, was with me as she usually is when I visit our cupboard. She seemed to be quite happy with what I was getting out. I know she likes tuna. She usually gets the first bite before I doctor it up. I was just about to open the can of tuna with the electric can opener when I noticed that the side of the can said "9 Lives Tuna Select." No wonder Noel was so happy. She thought I was giving her a can of one of her favorite treats.

Sometimes I don't take the time to really look and see what I'm looking at. Do you know what I mean? The cans are exactly the same size and tuna is written on both cans. Almost....

so close....a little too close if you ask me. I need to take more time to focus in on things. A mere look is not good enough. Oh well. Just another exciting moment in the life of one with Alzheimer's.

June 5, 2001

I decided to trim my hedges. Due to all the rain that we have been having here in Ohio, the hedges were looking like they needed a trim. I had about half of the hedge done and was feeling rather good about it. I was really pushing myself to get the rest done when all of a sudden I took a nice gash out of my finger with the trimmer. Ouch! Now to get the blood flow under control and also to sit down because I had gotten overheated while trying to finish my task, and I was feeling like I had better stop and sit down, or else.

Thinking back on the incident, I in no way should have hedge trimmers in my hands. I can think of many reasons. The main reason is that I am dangerous. I don't always see what is before me, and I can no longer measure distances with my eyes. My rate of thinking and responding has slowed down considerably, and I have poor judgment.

Although I know these things about myself, I still make poor decisions in projects I do around the home. There are always other ways to get the jobs accomplished, however. I have decided to look into getting outside help to trim the hedges the next time. By making plans ahead of time with the help of my wife, Sharon, I will not feel the need to get out there and do it myself. This is so important in keeping me out of trouble. I've decided that it is worth the time and effort.

June 10, 2001

I am not ashamed of having early-onset Alzheimer's Disease. Why should I be? I did not ask for the disease, or do anything to cause it. What do I have to be ashamed of? Why hide the fact that I have dementia? I am not proud of the fact, but neither am I ashamed of the fact. The certainty of the matter is that it is a fact and therefore I will share that fact. I do not fixate on it, or give it my whole life, although it will take my whole life in time.

But this is something that has happened to me and is a reality in my life every moment of every day, I feel I have every right to explore it openly, to share it, and to deal with it in whatever way I choose.

There are some that I know that deal with it privately and I give them that right. I deal with my disease openly and find it to be very healthy for me, even resulting in some healing for me. I share because it is good for me, and I hope that my sharing touches many other lives.

No, I am not ashamed that I have a disease called Alzheimer's. I have yet many miles to travel, and by sharing, those miles will be more blessed than by being silent.

June 20, 2001

I forgot to tell you. Soon I will have a new ID bracelet to wear. It's on order. Now when I get lost I will be returned to my home. How nice! I must admit that I have been lost a time or so. Got confused as to which way to turn and where I was. It all looked the same to me.

In our recent support meeting in Akron they discussed the Safe Return Program. Immediately my feathers were ruffled. Pride, I guess. I didn't need such a thing. I'm not at that stage yet. I don't wander. I'm seldom out by myself. I don't drive anymore. I've never been lost more than a few minutes.

I don't like bracelets. They don't come in my color—gold.

Sharon thought I needed one. After a little consideration, I finally agreed. I guess there are moments when I am out and about by myself when this program could give me assurance. Make me feel safe.

I can't promise that I'll wear it all the time, but I will wear it when I am out by myself. When I forget my address and phone number, which I sometimes do, I'll be returned to my home if I get lost.

June 23, 2001

I just finished the book *Show Me the Way to Go Home* by Larry Rose. What an exciting account of someone who has Alzheimer's Disease. Larry was 54 when he was diagnosed. I highly recommend the book. It's easy to read and tells us the feelings and events that one has with the disease.

This is the third book that I have read now by authors that have or had early stages of Alzheimer's Disease. The other two books were by Diana McGowin and Robert Davis. There are more and more books out there for individuals who are caregivers, family, or friends, but very few by someone who is affected by AD. I enjoy reading how others feel and what they have been through because of the disease.

I hope that more of us write books telling how it is. Others need to hear, and we need to write. The more I write the better I feel.

June 27, 2001

Today I had a tour of a large Alzheimer's Specialty Care Center.

There were six units, which can handle a total of 150 residents. Unit A was late beginning to early middle stage. Unit B, beginning stages, Unit C, safe haven for the wandering residents in the middle stages. Unit D was transitional middle stages, when social inappropriate behaviors can be present. Unit E was late middle and early end stage and Unit F was end stage for Alzheimer's Disease.

No matter how I tried, I didn't like what I saw. It seemed so void of life. Individuals being warehoused, waiting for the end. I told

Sharon not to take me to this particular place. I've been to several other locations and I have never seen this before. How very, very sad.

Perhaps I should not put myself through things like this. I guess I want to know what's out there. What could lie ahead? I must say that I have been to several places that I would not mind living in if needed, should the need present itself. I am not against them and feel that they are needed in many situations. I just have to work through what I saw today. That's all.

July 1, 2001

There was a time not long ago that I could do many things at once, and prided myself in being able to do so. I could go into my office, answer the phone, know what was going on in the office, carry on a conversation with my neighbor and take notes all at the same time. No more.

I was listening to CNN for news recently. My problem was that on the bottom of the screen was another small screen going the whole way across the bottom. It also had news on it and was moving quickly and constantly. After trying to concentrate on both the top and the bottom screen, I soon gave up in frustration. There's no way I could do both.

I noticed something while riding down the road with the radio on. Now I can do it with background music on very low, but I begin getting irritated when there are words to the music. It seems I can no longer ride in the car and listen to music with words at the same time. This is two things at once calling for my attention, and I just can't do it. I noticed that I don't do too well on chat lines when there are many chatters. I can't keep up and soon become overwhelmed.

I can only do one thing at a time well. Two things are questionable, and three things are out of the question. I'm sorry, but this is how I am becoming. That means one conversation at a time.

Please. I'm sure I will notice other changes in this area as time goes on. I'm not looking forward to them.

July 24, 2001

There are times in our house that things seem to disappear. Like today, Sharon was going to make me a glass of lemonade. How nice! And the next thing I knew she accused me of hiding the lemon juicer. Why...the nerve! It wasn't me, I said. Of course I didn't do it. Had nothing to do with it at all.

But then again, thinking about it a little more realistically for a moment, perhaps I did have something to do with it. See, I put the clean dry dishes away and this could have included a lemon juicer. I'm not admitting to anything, but it could have been me. I don't always put things back exactly where they belong. And there have been a few times that things have been discovered where they aren't usually kept. If I recall, there have been a few times we've had this problem when putting away the clean laundry.

Eventually the missing items do surface, but we may have to do without some things in the mean time. How am I to know where I store it? I only put it away, that's all. Go figure!

August 10, 2001

Recently before a large audience here at the National Hall of Fame's first football game of the season, a well-known singer was singing our National Anthem and forgot some of the words. She was booed and yelled at and only a few applauded her performance when it was over. She later said that she felt awful about what had happened, but she just all of a sudden had a mental block. She couldn't help it. It just happened. She and her backup group had practiced minutes before the performance with no problems at all, and she knew the words by heart, but it happened.

I can understand and sympathize with her. On occasion I am talking and I forget the words. They are not there and will not come. I forget what I was saying or forget the answer. I occasionally repeat myself.

When I first started repeating myself, I realized what I had been doing and tried to fix it. I became very careful about what I said. I became very conscious when I was conversing with others. I remember I was trying to relate with a new couple, when the wife looked at me and said, "You already said that." I felt so bad and embarrassed. I didn't know what to say.

Fortunately, most people are more gracious. They don't boo me, they don't give me that condescending look, they don't try to correct me. They go on as if it didn't happen. When I stop in the midst of a sentence, they seem to understand, and we go right on with our conversation. When things like this happen I do my best to cover it up, but there are many times when I am embarrassed by what happened. And I know it will happen again and more often as time goes on.

August 14, 2001

I feel I accomplished nothing today. I made it through the day. Wasn't that enough? Not really. I got out of bed, took care of myself, made myself some cereal for breakfast, and tuna for lunch. Read the paper, picked up some trash outside, and went to the library for two hours. But it just doesn't seem to be enough. I accomplished little, but I did make it through the day. Some days are like that. I guess I can consider that an accomplishment. I made it through another day. I would rather make it than not make it and that is my choice at the moment. It is a choice that I make daily. I'm thankful that I still have choice and that it is not one of the many losses I have experienced.

It's okay if I just make it through the day when that is all that I can do.

Tomorrow might be better, and many times tomorrow is better. It's never the way it used to be, but it can be better than today and that's what I am hoping for. That tomorrow is better than today. Day by day, moment by moment.

November 4, 2001

I was just wondering whether I block out certain things, and if I do, why? There are places in Alzheimer's Disease that I don't want to go. I have said before that I don't want to hurry the stages. I've read about the stages, had classes about the stages, and once was enough. It's a scary place to go.

So....why even go there the first time? I'm curious. I want to know what could happen to me. I need to know what to expect, how to prepare. Having said that, I've spent little time thinking about the latter stages. I have not planned well for that time in my life. Yes, Sharon and I have a power of attorney in place and I have a plot ready for the end of life. I have discussed nursing home placement if needed. But the details that can change—I don't want to go there.

Perhaps I will never get there—to the latter stages. Something gets us many times before we ever get there. For now, I won't go near there. I'm working on the Alzheimer's Disease diagnosis, living moment by moment in the present, not the future. I choose to stay in the moment at the moment. But I do want to think about the hope of a cure that might be right around the corner.

November 13, 2001

Well, been thinking about it for a long time now and I have decided it was time to do it. I need to cut back, way back on what we do with our time. It's not been easy to decide what gets cut back. My wife, Sharon, and I have discussed this situation over and over and I think we've come up with some things that will help us out.

We've decided to discontinue heading up the food program at our church. We will still volunteer when we are able. This was a difficult decision because we love the food program and feel it plays such an important purpose in our church and community.

I then decided that I would no longer work at qualifying for my social worker's license with the state of Ohio. The license means a lot to me and I have had it since the state began licensing. This means that I will no longer have to attend classes to meet the qualifications. I will still attend classes, but fewer, and of my choosing. I've also decided that I will no longer do public speaking. My voice no longer cooperates with me and this is another way that I can have more time for necessary things in my life.

I'm hoping by giving up these three things in my life that it will give us more time for much needed R&R.

SHARON'S TURN

Serving as her husband's caregiver for the last eight years has been hard on Sharon. The 58-year-old retired bookkeeper suffers from fibromyalgia and always expected Chip to be the one to take care of her, not the other way around. "I always thought my husband would be there to help take care of me, to run the vacuum, to run the errands or do whatever needed to be done," says Sharon. "But I haven't had a husband for four years."

The couple met as teenagers at a church youth camp. "I wanted him to ask me to a banquet so bad, and he did," she recalls. "He came to our church on a Wednesday night in July, 1965, and that's when we started going together." The following year, Chip went away to college and worked weekends in a psychiatric hospital. They saw each other one weekend a month, then got married in August 1966 and raised two daughters.

When Chip was first diagnosed with Alzheimer's, it was easy to deny it. Most times, he seemed perfectly fine. "But then he'd do something, and we'd say, 'Yup, he has Alzheimer's,'" she recalls.

Sharon admits she is frequently frustrated. Chip needs constant supervision with even the simplest tasks, like replacing a light bulb, and has the persistence of a small child when he wants something. At dinnertime, she waits on him hand and foot, while he asks her to retrieve his drink, his napkin, and whatever else he might need.

At times, Sharon says, she has to work to keep from yelling at him, but always tries to hold back and keep in mind that it is the disease that causes his behavior, his relentless requests, and his inability to deal with reality. "I have to remind myself that okay, I don't like this," she says. "I don't like it that I'm the one who always has to do the driving and the one who has to do everything. But I'm not the one who is losing my life. My feelings and actions should be more sympathetic toward him."

Although Chip's behavior is becoming increasingly childlike, Sharon says she has to resist the urge to treat him like a child. Rather than tell him what he can or can't do, Sharon looks for ways to lead him toward good decisions, so he thinks that he made the choice.

For instance, on Sundays after church, he sometimes asks to go out in the afternoon. But given that there's a potluck dinner that night, Sharon knows he'll be tired if they do. Rather than tell him no, she asks him, "Are you sure that's what you want to do? Do you really want to do this?" Sharon says that after some prodding, Chip will usually agree that she's right and that he's too tired.

Already this winter, he has been talking about going camping next summer. "In reality, he can't stand the heat," Sharon says. "And when he has to lie down, where is his couch going to be? The truth is, he's beyond camping. I know it, but he doesn't know it. But I just have to let him talk about it."

In the last two years, Sharon has seen Chip deteriorate considerably. Once a lover of family Christmas gatherings, he can no longer tolerate the noise and confusion created by his grandchildren, and wants to go to someone else's house so he can leave when he's ready. In the car, he can no longer stand to listen to music. The fatigue has worsened, and Chip has cut back considerably on his journaling.

His ability to sleep well has eroded, too. Frequent nightmares cause him to call out at night, and he awakens at the slightest noise. "In one of his dreams, two of our grandchildren are on fire, and he tries to beat the flames out," Sharon says. "He has people coming at him with knives and snakes trying to get him. He once literally jumped out of bed."

To help her cope, Sharon takes an anti-depressant. She also participates in a support group on the Internet, and she and Chip attend a support group twice a month. Some members have lost their spouses already, and others have spouses in the late stages. Hearing horror stories about spouses who urinate in trash cans or who have been kicked out of nursing homes is worrisome, but Sharon does not want to be blindsided by what might come. "I'm always waiting for the other shoe to drop," she says. "But I would rather know. If some of these things don't happen, then I got lucky."

RESOURCES

If you were recently diagnosed with early Alzheimer's, you are probably trying to learn as much as you can about the disease. Whether it's finding a good support group in your area, reading the experiences of others who have the disease, or getting information on financial matters, there is a wealth of information available—in your library, on the Internet, and through local, state, and national organizations that deal with Alzheimer's.

We've provided a list of some of the best sources of information. Though the list consists of some of the best, it is by no means comprehensive. Instead, these organizations, books, and Web sites may lead you to other resources as you slowly build your knowledge of the disease.

Alzheimer's Association
225 North Michigan Avenue
17th Floor
Chicago, IL 60601-7633
Tel: 312-335-8700 or 1-800-272-3900
Fax: 312-335-1110
Online: http://www.alz.org
E-mail: info@alz.org

The Alzheimer's Association is the world leader in Alzheimer's re-search and support, and the largest and oldest volunteer organization dedicated to the prevention, treatment, care, and support of AD.

It also offers the Safe Return program for patients with Alzheimer's who wander and become lost. For a one-time $40 fee, participants can get the aid of community support network, in-cluding local law enforcement. To enroll, contact 1-888-572-8566.

Alzheimer's Disease Education and Referral Center (ADEAR)
P.O. Box 8250
Silver Spring, MD 20907-8250
Tel: 301-495-3311 or 1-800-438-4380
Fax: 301-495-3334
Online: http://www.alzheimers.org
E-mail: adear@alzheimers.org

The Alzheimer's Disease Education and Referral (ADEAR) Center was created in 1990 to "compile, archive, and disseminate information concerning Alzheimer's disease" for health professionals, people with AD and their families, and the public. It is operated as a service of the National Institute on Aging (NIA), which is a branch of the National Institutes of Health and part of the U.S. Department of Health and Human Services.

According to its Web site, the ADEAR Center "strives to be a current, comprehensive, unbiased source of information about AD. All our information and materials about the search for causes, treatment, cures, and better diagnostic tools are carefully researched and thoroughly reviewed by NIA scientists and health communicators for accuracy and integrity."

Alzheimer's Foundation of America
322 Eighth Avenue
6th Floor
New York, NY 10001
Tel: 1-866-AFA-8484 (232-8484)
Fax: 1-516-767-6864
Online: http://www.alzfdn.org
E-mail: info@alzfdn.org

Founded in 2002, the Alzheimer's Foundation of America is a non-profit foundation comprised of member and associate member organizations across the United States committed to meeting the educational, social, and emotional needs of individuals with Alzheimer's disease and their families and caregivers. The organization works to promote public awareness of the disease and provides expertise to healthcare professionals. Its mission is "to provide optimal care and services to individuals confronting dementia and to their caregivers and families through member organizations dedicated to improving quality of life."

Alzinfo.org
Fisher Center for Alzheimer's Research Foundation
One Intrepid Square
West 46th Street and 12th Avenue
New York, NY 10036
Tel: 1-800-ALZINFO
Online: www.alzinfo.org

Alzinfo.org was created by the Fisher Center for Alzheimer's Research Foundation as a way to educate people about this disease. The Web site also provides an online community with continuous access to information and support through online chats, message boards, and some of the most comprehensive resource databases available on the topic.

The Fisher Center for Alzheimer's Research Foundation is a nonprofit founded in 1995 to gather information on the cause, care, and cure of Alzheimer's disease according to criteria set by the National Institutes of Health.

American Health Assistance Foundation

22512 Gateway Center Drive
Clarksburg, MD 20871
Tel: 1-800-437-AHAF (2423)
Fax: 301-258-9454
Online: http://www.ahaf.org
E-mail: info@ahaf.org

Since 1985, the American Health Assistance foundation has operated the Alzheimer's Disease Research (ADR) program, which
funds research on and educates the public about Alzheimer's disease. Since its inception, ADR has awarded more than $40.3 mil-
lion to support promising research in fields ranging from
molecular biology to epidemiology.

Family Caregiver Alliance

180 Montgomery Street
Suite 1100
San Francisco, CA 94104
Tel: 1-800-445-8106
Fax: 415-434-3508
Online: http://www.caregiver.org
E-mail: info@caregiver.org

The Family Caregiver Alliance was founded in 1977, and was the
first community-based nonprofit organization in the country to
address the needs of families and friends providing long-term care
at home. FCA offers numerous programs in education and support
for people in the throes of caregiving and is also involved in advocacy work to address caregiver needs in public policy. The group
operates at national, state, and local levels to support and sustain
caregivers.

Other organizations that might be of interest to persons with Alzheimer's and their families include the following:

FOR CAREGIVERS AND PATIENTS

Administration on Aging
Washington, DC 20201
Tel: 202-619-0724
Fax: 202-357-3555
Online: http://www.aoa.gov

AlzOnline.Net
Tel: 1-866-260-2466
Online: www.alzonline.net
E-mail: info@alzonline.net

Children of Aging Parents
P.O. Box 167
Richboro, PA 18954
Tel: 1-800-227-7294
Online: http://www.caps4caregivers.org

C-Mac Informational Services/Caregiver News
120 Clinton Lane
Cookeville, TN 38501-8946
Online: http://www.caregivernews.org
E-mail: caregiver_cmi@hotmail.com

Dementia Advocacy and Support Network International
P.O. Box 1645
Mariposa, CA 95338
Online: http://www.dasninternational.org

National Council on the Aging
300 D Street, SW
Suite 801
Washington, D.C. 20024
Tel: 202-479-1200
Fax: 202-479-0735
Online: http://www.ncoa.org
E-mail: info@ncoa.org

National Family Caregivers Association
10400 Connecticut Avenue
Suite 500
Kensington, MD 20895-3944
Tel: 301-942-6430 or 1-800-896-3650
Fax: 301-942-2302
Online: http://www.nfcacares.org
E-mail: info@nfcacares.org

Medline Plus
http://www.nlm.nih.gov/medlineplus/alzheimersdisease.html

National Respite Network and Resource Center
800 Eastowne Drive
Suite 105
Chapel Hill, NC 27514
Tel: 919-490-5577 or 1-800-7-RELIEF (773-5433)
Fax: 919-490-4905
Online: http://www.archrespite.org

Well Spouse Foundation
63 West Main Street, Suite H
Freehold, NJ 07728
Tel: 732-577-8899 or 1-800-838-0879
Fax: 732-577-8644
Online: http://www.wellspouse.org
E-mail: info@wellspouse.org

FOR FUTURE PLANNING
Aging With Dignity
P.O. Box 1661
Tallahassee, FL 32301-1661
Tel: 1-888-5-WISHES (1-888-594-7437)
Online: www.agingwithdignity.org

American Association of Homes and Services for the Aging
2519 Connecticut Avenue, NW
Washington, DC 20008
Tel: 1-202-783-2242
Fax: 1-202-783-2255
Online: http://www.aahsa.org

Assisted Living Federation of America
11200 Waples Mill Rd, #150
Fairfax, VA 22030
Tel: 1-703-691-8100
Fax: 1-703-691-8106
Online: http://www.alfa.org
E-mail: info@alfa.org

Centers for Medicare and Medicaid Services
7500 Security Boulevard
Baltimore, MD 21244-1850
Tel: 1-877-267-2323
Online: http://www.cms.hhs.gov

The Eldercare Locator
Tel: 1-800-677-1116
Online: http://www.eldercare.gov

Financial Planners Association
4100 E. Mississippi Ave.
Suite 400
Denver, CO 80246-3053
Tel: 1-800-322-4237
Fax: 303-759-0749
Online: http://www.fpanet.org

National Citizens' Coalition for Nursing Home Reform
801 L Street, NW
Suite 801
Washington, DC 20036
Tel: 202-332-2275
Fax: 202-332-2949
Online: http://www.nursinghomeaction.org

National Academy of Elder Law Attorneys, Inc.
1604 North Country Club Rd.
Tucson, AZ 85716
Tel: 520-881-4005
Fax: 520-325-7925
Online: http://www.naela.org

Social Security Administration
Office of Public Inquiries
Windsor Park Building
6401 Security Blvd.
Baltimore, MD 21235
Tel: 1-800-772-1213
Online: http://www.ssa.gov

RESEARCH
American Federation for Aging Research
70 West 40th St., 11th floor
New York, NY 10018
Tel: 212-703-9977 or 1-888-582-2327
Fax: 212-997-0330
Online: http://www.afar.org and http://www.infoaging.org
E-mail: grants@afar.org or info@afar.org

Clinicaltrials.gov
http://www.clinicaltrials.gov

Institute for the Study of Aging
1414 Avenue of the Americas
Suite 1502
New York, NY 10019
Tel: 212-935-2402
Fax: 212-935-2408
Online: http://www.aging-institute.org
E-mail: hfillit@aging-institute.org

National Institute on Aging
Building 31, Room 5C27
31 Center Drive, MSC 2292
Bethesda, MD 20892
Online: http://www.nia.nih.gov

National Institutes of Health (NIH)
9000 Rockville Pike
Bethesda, MD 20892
Tel: 301-496-4000 (Other toll-free NIH
telephone numbers can be found online.)
Online: http://www.nih.gov/health/infoline.htm.

OTHER ORGANIZATIONS OF INTEREST
American Association of Retired Persons
601 E. Street NW
Washington, DC 20049
Tel: 1-888-OUR-AARP (1-888-687-2277)
Online: http://www.aarp.org

American Diabetes Association
ATTN: National Call Center
1701 North Beauregard Street
Alexandria, VA 22311
Tel: 1-800-342-2383
Online: http://www.diabetes.org

American Heart Association
National Center
7272 Greenville Avenue
Dallas, TX 75231
Tel: AHA: 1-800-AHA-USA-1 or 1-800-242-8721
Online: http://www.americanheart.org

American Stroke Association
National Center
7272 Greenville Avenue
Dallas TX 75231
Tel: 1-888-4-STROKE or 1-888-478-7653
Online: http://www.americanstroke.org

Faith in Action
Wake Forest University School of Medicine
Medical Center Boulevard
Winston-Salem, NC 27157-1204
Tel: 1-877-324-8411
Fax: 336-716-3346
Online: http://www.fiavolunteers.org
E-mail: fia@wfubmc.edu

Mayo Clinic
http://www.mayoclinic.com

National Association for Continence
P.O. Box 1019
Charleston, SC 29402-1019
Phone: 1-800-BLADDER (252-3337)
Fax: 843-377-0905
Online: http://www.nafc.org
E-mail: memberservices@nafc.org

National Institute of Neurological Disorders and Stroke
NIH Neurological Institute
P.O. Box 5801
Bethesda, MD 20824
Tel: 1-800-352-9424
Online: http://www.ninds.nih.gov

National Organization for Rare Disorders (NORD)
P.O. Box 1968
55 Kenosia Avenue
Danbury, CT 06813-1968
Tel: 1-800-999-NORD (6673)
Fax: 203-798-2291
Online: http://www.rarediseases.org
E-mail: orphan@rarediseases.org

National Institute of Mental Health (NIMH)
National Institutes of Health, DHHS
6001 Executive Blvd. Rm. 8184, MSC 9663
Bethesda, MD 20892-9663
Tel: 301-443-4513 or 301-443-8431
Fax: 301-443-4279
Online: http://www.nimh.nih.gov
E-Mail: nimhinfo@nih.gov

**National Hospice and Palliative Care Organization/
National Hospice Foundation**
1700 Diagonal Road
Suite 625
Alexandria, VA 22314
Tel: 1-800-658-8898
Fax: 703-837-1233
Online: http://www.nhpco.org
E-mail: nhpco_info@nhpco.org

National Sleep Foundation
1522 K Street, NW, Suite 500
Washington, DC 20005
Tel: 202-347-3471
Fax: 202-347-3472
Online: http://www.nsf.org
E-mail: nsf@sleepfoundation.org

U.S. Food and Drug Administration
5600 Fishers Lane
Rockville, MD 20857-0001
Tel: 1-888-INFO-FDA (1-888-463-6332)
Online: http://www.fda.gov

BOOKS FOR ADULTS

Alzheimer's Early Stages: First Steps for Family, Friends and Caregivers, by Daniel Kuhn (Hunter House, 2003).

The Alzheimer's Healthcare Handbook, by Mary S. Mittelman, Dr., Ph., and Cynthia Epstein, ACSW (Marlowe & Co., 2002).

Developing Support Groups for Individuals with Early-Stage Alzheimer's Disease: Planning, Implementation and Evaluation, by Robyn Yale, LCSW (Health Professions Press, 1995).

The Forgetting: Alzheimer's, Portrait of an Epidemic, by David Shenk, (Anchor Books, 2003).

Just Love Me, My Life Turned Upside Down by Alzheimer's, by Jeanne L. Lee (Purdue University Press, 2003).

Living in the Labyrinth: A Personal Journey Through the Maze of Alzheimer's, by Diana McGowin (Delta Books, 1994).

Mayo Clinic on Alzheimer's Disease, edited by Ronald Petersen, MD., PhD. (Mayo Clinic Health Information, 2002).

Preventing Alzheimer's: Ways to Help Prevent, Delay, Detect, and Even Halt Alzheimer's Disease and Other Forms of Memory Loss, by William Rodman Shankle, M.S., M.D. and Daniel Amen, M.D. (GP Putnam's, 2004).

Speaking Our Minds: Personal Reflections from Individuals with Alzheimer's, by Lisa Snyder (Henry Holt & Co., 2000).

There's Still a Person in There: The Complete Guide to Treating and Coping With Alzheimer's, by Michael Castleman, Dolores Gallagher-Thompson, Matthew Naythons (Putnam Publishing Group, 2000).

The 36-Hour Day: A Family Guide to Caring for Persons with Alzheimer Disease, Related Dementing Illnesses and Memory Loss in Later Life, by Nancy L. Mace, M.A. and Peter V. Rabin, M.D., MPh. (Johns Hopkins University Press, 1999).

BOOKS FOR CHILDREN
Allie Learns about Alzheimer's Disease: A Family Story about Love, Patience and Acceptance, by Kim Gosselin (JayJo Books, 2002).

Alzheimer's Disease (Diseases and People), by Edward Willett (Enslow Publishers, 2002).

An Early Winter, by Marion Dane Bauer (Bantam Doubleday Dell Books for Young Readers, 1999).

Grandma's Cobwebs, by Ann Frantti (Dagney Publishing, 2002).

Horse Whispers in the Air, by Dandi Daley MacKall (Concordia Publishing House, 2000).

It Only Looks Easy, by Pamela Curtis Swallow (Mill Brook Press, 2003).

Remember Me? Alzheimer's Through the Eyes of a Child (Te Acuerdas de Mi?), by Sue Glass (Raven Tree Press LLC, 2002).

Singing with Momma Lou, by Linda Jacobs Altman (Lee and Low Books, Inc., 2002).

The Graduation of Jake Moon, by Barbara Park (Athenaeum Books for Young Readers, 2000).

The Stranger I Call Grandma: A Story About Alzheimer's Disease, by Swanee Ballman (Jawbone Publishing Corporation, 2001).

PHARMACEUTICAL COMPANY WEB SITES
http://aricept.com
http://www.exelon.com
http://www.memantine.com
http://www.us.reminyl.com

GLOSSARY

Acetylcholine: A chemical messenger in the brain that is involved in the formation of memories, thought, and judgment, and controlling muscle contractions and hormone secretion. In people with Alzheimer's, there is often lower levels of acetylcholine than that in healthy people.

Acetylcholinesterase: An enzyme that aids in the breakdown of acetylcholine.

Adult day centers: A place for Alzheimer's patients to go to engage in activities, such as arts and crafts, music, discussions, and support groups.

Agitation: A category of troubling behaviors that often occur in Alzheimer's, and in the early stages may include irritability, anxiety, or depression.

Agnosia: A condition in which a person has trouble using information gathered from his senses.

Alzheimer's disease: An irreversible age-related form of dementia that slowly erodes the brain. It robs the person of memory and cognitive skills, and causes changes in personality and behavior.

Alzheimer's Disease Neuroimaging Initiative: A five-year collaborative effort by the National Institute on Aging and several other agencies, private companies, and organizations to study changes in the brain that suggest the development of Alzheimer's and can be detected by neuroimaging techniques such as serial magnetic resonance imaging (MRI) and positron emission tomography (PET). Scientists will also be examining other biological markers for clues.

Alzhemed: An experimental drug for the treatment of Alzheimer's that works by binding to beta amyloid in the brain before plaques can form. It also helps to remove beta amyloid from the brain and blocks the inflammatory process associated with amyloid buildup in the disease process.

Ampalex: An experimental drug also known as CX516 that may improve the symptoms of Alzheimer's by aiding the attachment of glutamate to special receptor cells. Glutamate is an amino acid and chemical messenger released by brain cells that plays a pivotal role in information processing, storage, and memory.

Amygdala: A part of the limbic system of the brain that houses the body's fight or flight response system and governs powerful emotions such as fear and anger.

Amyloid β-diffusible ligands (ADDL): A type of protein that is present in cerebral spinal fluid at a very low concentration in early stage Alzheimer's. ADDLs are only five nanometers wide.

Amyloid precursor protein (APP): A substance believed to play a role in the growth and survival of neurons. When APP gets lodged between the inside and outside of a cell membrane, it is clipped by enzymes.

Anticonvulsants: Medications used to treat seizures and stabilize moods.

Antipsychotics: Medications used to treat hallucinations, delusions, aggression, and hostility. It may also be prescribed for insomnia.

Anxiolytic: A medication used to treat anxiety.

Anxiety: A mental disorder characterized by persistent distress that is common among people with Alzheimer's.

Aphasia: A condition characterized by difficulty with communication. Losing the ability to speak and write is called expressive aphasia, while the inability to understand spoken or written words is called receptive aphasia.

Apolipoprotein E: A gene that is responsible for the transport of cholesterol in the blood. The APOE gene has three naturally occurring variants, or alleles, epsilon-2, epsilon-3, and epsilon-4. Carrying one or two variants of epsilon- 4 increases the chances that you'll develop late-onset AD.

Apolipoprotein E epsilon-4 (APOE-4): A gene whose variant has been linked to a greater likelihood of developing late-onset Alzheimer's. Scientists believe that APOE epsilon-4 is less effective at dissolving beta amyloid from the brain than the other alleles.

APP gene: A gene responsible for making APP, the membrane protein that gets lodged between the inside and outside of the cell on chromosome 21. The mutations associated with Alzheimer's occur on the part of the APP that's sticking out of the cell, which causes the formation of excess beta amyloid plaques.

Assisted living: A residential facility for older adults who can live somewhat independently but still need some assistance in day-to-day care or medical care. Also called board and care, group homes, community-based residential facilities, or foster homes.

Benzodiazepines: A class of drugs commonly prescribed to cause sedation, induce sleep, relieve anxiety, eliminate muscle spasms, and prevent seizures.

Beta amyloid: A protein fragment that has been snipped from a larger protein called (APP), a substance believed to play a role in the growth and survival of neurons. These protein fragments are less soluble and stickier, and when they cluster together the process of plaque formation begins.

Beta amyloid plaques: Sticky deposits made up primarily of beta amyloid, but which also contains other proteins, neuron remnants, and immune cells known as microglia. The plaques are a key feature of Alzheimer's disease and believed to be responsible for the cognitive decline that occurs.

Beta secretase: An enzyme involved in the cleaving of amyloid precursor protein (APP) that leads to the production of beta amyloid. Inhibition of this enzyme, which could potentially slow or prevent the formation of plaques, is being studied as a possible treatment for Alzheimer's.

Binswanger's disease: A rare form of dementia sometimes called subcortical dementia that is characterized by cerebrovascular lesions in the deep white matter of the brain.

Bio-barcode amplification: An emerging technology that is being developed to measure the presence of protein amyloid β-diffusible ligands, or ADDLs in cerebrospinal fluid.

Board certification: A level of expertise achieved by a medical doctor who has trained rigorously in his medical specialty and passed an exam that tests his knowledge.

Body Mass Index: A measure of weight in relation to height. To calculate BMI, multiply your weight in pounds by 703. Divide that number by your height in inches, squared (i.e., height x height).

Brain stem: A part of the brain that sits at the base and connects the spinal cord to the brain. The brain stem, which is the smallest part of the brain, controls our body's autonomic processes, such as our heart rate and breathing. It also controls sleep and dreaming.

Cardiovascular disease: A category of medical conditions that result in damage to blood vessels supplying blood to the heart. Studies suggest that cardiovascular disease may be linked to Alzheimer's.

Caregiver: Anyone who cares for the needs of another person either temporarily or permanently.

Central nervous system: The part of the nervous system made up of the brain and spinal cord that is responsible for receiving information from inside and outside the body, then relaying the information to the brain to determine the correct response.

Cerebellum: A part of the brain comprised of two hemispheres that coordinates balance and movement.

Cerebral cortex: The outer layer of the cerebrum where higher brain functions take place. It is here that the brain processes the barrage of sensory information it receives, controls our movements, and regulates thoughts and mental activity.

Cerebrovascular disease: A condition characterized by clots in the small blood vessels that supply blood to the brain, causing problems in blood flow that may lead to vascular dementia.

Cerebrum: The largest part of the brain that is made up of the right and left hemispheres. The cerebrum contains your gray matter, which gives its outside surface a grayish-brown hue. It is the center of most of your cognitive processes. Efforts like thinking, analyzing, organizing, and decision-making in large part take place here.

Cholinesterase inhibitors: A class of medications used to treat Alzheimer's that slow the breakdown of acetylcholine and can help lessen the symptoms of Alzheimer's.

Clinical trials: Carefully conducted research studies done in human volunteers to answer specific questions about a treatment, vaccine, medical device or procedure. The trials are done to find out how the new therapy or procedure will work in people, and to determine its risks and its effectiveness.

Computerized tomography: A type of imaging technology that shoots two dimensional images of a body part or organ. Also known as a CT scan.

Continuing care retirement community (CCRC): A campus-like residential community that features a spectrum of senior housing ranging from independent retirement homes to nursing home facilities.

Corpus callosum: A thick band of nerve cell fibers located in the center of the two hemispheres that links all the billions of neurons.

C-reactive protein: A substance produced during the inflammatory process that has been linked to the development of Alzheimer's.

Creutzfeldt-Jakob disease: A contagious and fatal form of dementia that is caused by misshapen brain proteins called prions, which attack healthy brain tissue. A variant of CJD, which was contracted by eating tainted beef, caused an epidemic of mad cow disease in the 1990s.

Dementia: Any of a number of brain disorders that cause changes in the way your brain functions.

Dementia with Lewy bodies: A type of dementia characterized by the presence of Lewy bodies, small, round inclusions seen only upon autopsy in the brain stem and cortical regions of the brain. Symptoms resemble those seen in Alzheimer's.

Depression: A serious mood disorder and mental illness that is characterized by persistent sadness.

Disability insurance: A type of insurance coverage that is provided when a worker is no longer able to continue working.

Donepezil (Aricept): A cholinesterase inhibitor approved for the treatment of Alzheimer's. Approved by the FDA in 1996, donezepil has emerged as the most commonly prescribed cholinesterase inhibitor for the treatment of AD.

Do-not-resuscitate order: A document signed by a physician that directs that cardiopulmonary resuscitation (CPR) not be performed in the event it is required.

Down syndrome: A genetic disorder that results from an extra copy of chromosome 21. People with Down syndrome often have brain changes similar to those seen in people with Alzheimer's.

Durable power of attorney (DPA): A person you appoint to act on your behalf when you can no longer make any decisions yourself. The DPA is typically a trusted family member who knows you quite well and who ultimately becomes fully responsible for all decisions regarding your welfare, including medical and financial matters.

Enzyme-linked immunoassays: Diagnostic tests commonly known as the ELISA tests, which are used to detect the presence of antibodies.

Fibrillar beta-amyloid aggregates: Clusters of oligomers that ultimately become beta amyloid plaques.

Flurbiprofen (Flurizan): A type of non-steroidal anti-inflammatory drug that is being tested as a way to slow the progression of Alzheimer's.

Folate: A type of B vitamin that may help reduce levels of homocysteine in the blood and lower the risk for Alzheimer's.

Frontal lobe: A part of the brain located just behind your forehead that is largely responsible for your personality and which also handles problem solving, abstract thinking, and skilled movement.

Galantamine (Reminyl): The newest cholesterinase inhibitor on the market. In early 2005, the safety of galantamine was questioned after two studies on the drug's effects on mild cognitive impairment found that more patients taking the drug had died than those who were taking a placebo.

Gamma-aminobutyric acid (GABA): A chemical messenger in the brain that relays information back and forth from the sensory organs such as the eyes, back to the brain. Scientists have found that a lack of GABA can lead to the cognitive decline associated with Alzheimer's.

Gamma secretase: An enzyme involved in the cleaving of amyloid precursor protein (APP) that leads to the production of beta amyloid. Inhibition of this enzyme, which could potentially slow or prevent the formation of plaques, is being studied as a possible treatment for Alzheimer's.

Geriatricians: Medical doctors trained in the treatment of older patients, typically people older than age 65.

Gingko biloba: An herbal remedy derived from an ancient Chinese tree that scientists suspect may improve memory and slow the progression of dementia. Gingko may work by increasing blood flow in the brain and boosting neurotransmitter activity.

Glutamate: A neurotransmitter in the brain that plays a vital role in the abilities to process, store, and retrieve information. People who have Alzheimer's are believed to have excess glutamate.

Healthcare proxy (HCP): A legal document in which you appoint an agent to make healthcare decisions for you in the event you become incapacitated.

Hippocampus: A part of the limbic system in the brain that regulates your ability to memorize, store, sort, and retrieve information. Scientists believe the hippocampus is the site where short-term memories are converted into long-term memories and sent to be stored elsewhere in the brain.

Hormonal disorders: Disorders involving the organs that secrete or regulate hormones, chemical messengers that help regulate bodily functions, including reproduction, metabolism, and growth. These disorders can bring on symptoms of dementia.

Huntington's disease: A degenerative brain disorder that involves the progressive wasting away of neurons. As the disease progresses, it may produce symptoms of dementia.

Huperzine A: An herbal supplement derived from the plant *Huperzia serrata* that is being tested as a treatment for Alzheimer's.

Hypothalamus: A part of the limbic system in the brain that controls hormones, food intake, and body temperature.

Inflammation: A response by the immune system to injuries and foreign invaders such as cuts, viruses, and disease that some experts believe may play a role in the development of Alzheimer's.

In-home care: An arrangement that involves a trained aide coming to your home to provide services for someone who is serving as caregiver to a person with a medical condition such as Alzheimer's. Services might include supervision, recreational activities, medical assistance, exercise, grooming, housekeeping, meal preparation, and shopping.

Late-onset Alzheimer's disease: The form of Alzheimer's that develops in patients who are older than age 65.

Leuprolide: A hormone medication prescribed to men who have prostate cancer and women who have endometriosis or uterine fibroids that is being studied as a treatment to slow the progress of Alzheimer's and improve cognitive function.

Limbic system: A region of the brain located at the center of cerebral hemispheres that governs emotions, instincts, and motivation. It connects the brain stem to regions of the cerebral cortex.

Living will: A legal document in which you express specific directions as to your wishes with respect to extraordinary measures and life-sustaining procedures such as life support.

Long-term care insurance: A type of insurance coverage that may help you cover the expenses involved in nursing home or extended care.

Lumbar puncture: A procedure commonly called a spinal tap that involves inserting a needle into the spinal canal and withdrawing cerebrospinal fluid for examination. Examining the cerebrospinal fluid that supports the brain can provide information about the presence of other diseases.

Magnetic resonance imaging: A type of imaging that uses magnetic fields and radio waves to pick up small energy signals emitted by the atoms that comprise body tissue, then produces images of organs and structures in the body. Also called an MRI.

Medicaid: A form of government assistance for people who have exhausted their resources. It may insure long-term care.

Medicare: The health insurance plan operated by the federal government that is available to most people over the age of 65. You may also be eligible for Medicare if you're under the age of 65 and have been on Social Security disability for at least twenty-four months.

Megaloblastic anemia: A condition caused by a vitamin B12 or folate deficiency that may resemble dementia.

Memantine: An N-methyl D-aspartate antagonist, or NMDA antagonist, that is believed to work by regulating levels of glutamate, a chemical messenger, or neurotransmitter, in the brain.

Metabolic disorders: Conditions that affect the way the body performs metabolic processes such as liver or pancreas disease, kidney or liver failure, hypoglycemia, or chemical imbalances. Such conditions can produce symptoms of dementia.

Microglia: Immune cells that surround and digest damaged cells or foreign substances that cause inflammation.

Microtubles: Support structures inside neurons that guide nutrients and molecules through the body of the cell.

Mild cognitive impairment: A condition characterized by minor memory or cognitive impairments but not severe enough for the diagnosis of Alzheimer's disease. People with MCI can think, reason, and carry on the daily activities of life without problem. Some people diagnosed with MCI go on to develop Alzheimer's, but others never do.

Mini-Mental State Exam (MMSE): A simple screening test used by doctors to gauge a patient's mental abilities, including memory, language, visual, spatial, and organizational skills. The test includes questions regarding your whereabouts and asks you to perform simple tasks.

Mutations: Unexpected changes in a single gene or in sections of chromosomes that can cause disease.

Nanometer: A unit of measurement that is one-billionth of a meter.

Nanoscale technology: A type of technology using tiny units of measurement that is being examined as a way to diagnose Alzheimer's at earlier stages.

Neramexane: An experimental drug that might help slow the progress of Alzheimer's and improve cognitive function in patients. The drug is an N-methyl-D-aspartate (NMDA) receptor antagonist, which works by regulating the activity of glutamate, a chemical messenger involved in information processing, storage, and retrieval.

Neurofibrillary tangles: A defining characteristic of the Alzheimer's brain that is comprised of proteins inside neurons called tau that have bound together. Scientists believe these tangles cause poor communication among nerve cells, and later on, can cause them to die.

Neurologists: Medical doctors trained in the study of the brain and nervous system.

Neurons: Nerve cells in the brain that continuously receive and process nerve impulses.

Neurotransmitters: Chemical messengers that are released in the presence of an impulse traveling across neurons.

NMDA antagonists: A class of medications used to treat Alzheimer's by regulating levels of glutamate, a neurotransmitter.

NMDA receptors: Channels located on nerve cells that regulate the amount of calcium that enters a nerve cell. If NMDA receptors allow too much calcium into a nerve cell, they can be damaged or destroyed.

Nonsteroidal anti-inflammatory drugs (NSAIDs): A class of medications that is commonly used to achieve relief from pain and swelling, and the reduction of fever. Scientists believe that some NSAIDs may lower the risk for Alzheimer's.

Normal pressure hydrocephalus (NPH): A condition caused by a buildup of cerebrospinal fluid that occurs when the flow of cerebrospinal fluid is blocked. It is commonly called "water on the brain," and can produce symptoms of dementia.

Nun Study: An ongoing research effort involving members of religious communities that has examined the effects of aging on the brain and the impact of lifestyle factors on the incidence of Alzheimer's.

Nursing homes: Residential facilities that offer round-the-clock health care for residents. Some may even have special units just for people who have dementia.

Occipital lobe: The part of the brain that interprets visual information. It is found behind each hemisphere.

Oligomers: Clusters of beta amyloid fragments that have become less soluble and promote the formation of fibrillar beta-amyloid aggregates which become plaques.

Omega-3 fatty acids: Healthy fats found in certain fish that have anti-inflammatory effects that not only lower the risk for cardiovascular disease but may keep Alzheimer's at bay.

Oxidative stress: Damage of body cells caused by excessive amounts of highly reactive molecules called free radicals.

Parietal lobe: The part of the brain just behind the frontal lobe where sensory information, such as taste, smells, and textures is received. It also helps you determine your location in space using visual and spatial cues and allows you to navigate your surroundings.

Peripheral nervous system: A vast network of nerves that extends from the spinal cord to the far reaches of the body, such as toes and fingertips.

Pick's disease: A rare form of dementia caused by tangles of tau protein in the brain that cause neurons to swell and produce symptoms such as a lack of coordination, the loss of language abilities, the inability to recognize familiar people, places, and objects, and a loss of inhibition. Considered a variety of frontotemporal dementia.

Pittsburgh Compound B: A substance being developed by scientists at the University of Pittsburgh that experts hope will enable doctors to detect the presence of Alzheimer's in someone's brain while the patient is still alive.

Presenilin genes: Genes responsible for the clipping of APP into plaque-producing fragments. More than thirty different mutations of these proteins can trigger early-onset AD. These mutations promote the production of a specific kind of beta amyloid that is stickier and more prone to producing plaques. Presenilin genes have a strong connection to familial forms of AD, in which the disease strikes several members of the same family.

Primary care physicians: Doctors trained in general medical care, who may specialize in family or internal medicine.

Psychiatrists: Medical doctors trained in the prevention, diagnosis and treatment of mental, addictive, and emotional disorders.

Respite care: A temporary source of care for a person with Alzheimer's or another disease that provides a caregiver with a break from the job. One example is adult day care.

Residential respite care: Overnight stays for the person who has dementia that provide the caregiver with a chance for an extended reprieve.

Retirement housing: A type of residential community for older adults who can live independently and have few health concerns. Also called senior apartments or senior living facilities.

Reverse mortgages: A type of home equity loan for someone over the age of 62 who owns a single-family home outright. A reverse mortgage allows you to convert some of the home equity into cash without requiring you to sell your home.

Rivastigmine (Exelon): A cholestinerase inhibitor that also inhibits butyrylcholinesterase, another enzyme involved in the breakdown of acetylcholine.

Selective serotonin reuptake inhibitors (SSRIs): A class of anti-depressant medications that may reduce depressive symptoms in patients with Alzheimer's by blocking the removal of serotonin, a neurotransmitter, in the synapses between the nerves.

SGS742: An experimental drug known as a GABA receptor antagonist that has been found in earlier trials to improve attention and memory.

Simvastatin: A statin medication that has been associated with a decreased incidence of Alzheimer's. The drug's ability to slow the progression of AD is being studied in a clinical trial involving patients with mild to moderate Alzheimer's.

Single photon emission computed tomography: A type of imaging technology, also called SPECT, that involves injecting a small amount of a radioactive substance into the body. The more blood flow there is in a particular organ, such as the brain, the more the substance is taken up. A camera takes pictures of the brain activity, which are then converted by computer into cross-sectional images and three-dimensional images.

Social Security Disability Income: A form of government assistance for people under age 65 who can prove they can no longer work, or that the condition will last at least a year or that it will result in death.

Social worker: A health care professional who is often trained to provide counseling and who is well-versed in the services a community provides.

Statins: A class of drugs commonly prescribed to lower cholesterol that may also reduce the risk for Alzheimer's disease.

Stroke: A medical emergency that occurs when the arteries supplying blood to the brain suffers a blockage or a leak, and the brain can't get the oxygen and glucose it needs to function. Studies suggest that people who have experienced strokes are more likely to develop Alzheimer's.

Subdural hematoma: A buildup of blood that occurs between the brain's outer covering and the surface of the brain, often brought on by a head injury. The buildup is usually the result of a ruptured blood vessel.

Supplemental Security Income: A type of government assistance for people aged 65 or older, disabled or blind, and who have very limited income and assets may be eligible to receive SSI. In order to receive SSI, you must meet the Social Security Administration's definition of disability.

Synapse: A gap between neurons where an impulse triggers the release of chemical messengers called neurotransmitters.

Tacrine (Cognex): The first cholestinerase inhibitor to receive FDA approval in 1993. Today it is rarely prescribed and no longer marketed because of its link to liver damage.

Tau: Proteins inside the neurons that help give neurons their structure by binding to support structures in the cell called microtubules. In a person with Alzheimer's, tau is changed chemically and instead of binding to microtubules, begins to bind to other tau, causing the microtubules to disintegrate.

Temporal lobe: The part of your brain responsible for hearing, some aspects of language comprehension, perception, and essential memory functions. It is located at the side of your forehead, just behind your temple.

Thalamus: A part of the brain that processes, prioritizes, and delivers sensory information to other parts of the brain.

Trans fatty acids: A type of fat commonly found in processed foods that are produced during the hydrogenation process. Manufacturers use hydrogenation to help extend the shelf life of a food.

Tricyclics: A category of anti-depressants that work by restoring chemical imbalances in the brain that can cause depression.

Valproate: An anticonvulsant drug used to treat seizures in epilepsy that is being studied as a possible treatment for agitation in Alzheimer's. The drug, which is also used to treat the manic phase of bipolar disorder and migraine headaches, may also slow the cognitive decline that occurs with Alzheimer's.

Vascular dementia: A type of dementia that results from a series of small strokes or changes in the arteries that supply blood to the brain. Also called multi-infarct dementia, it is the second most common kind of dementia. Symptoms include loss of intellectual abilities, difficulties with language, confusion, and problems following directions.

Viatical settlements: An investment vehicle that allows a terminally ill person to sell an existing life insurance policy to a third party in return for a percentage of the face value of the policy, which is paid immediately.

Vitamin B6: A type of B vitamin that helps reduce levels of homocysteine in the blood and lowers the risk for Alzheimer's.

Vitamin B12: A type of B vitamin that is often difficult to absorb in elderly people. Deficiencies of vitamin B12 can produce symptoms that resemble Alzheimer's. Vitamin B12 may also help reduce levels of homocysteine in the blood and lower the risk for Alzheimer's.

Vitamin C: An antioxidant vitamin with the potential for slowing the damage caused by free radicals. Good sources include red bell peppers, leafy greens, strawberries, and oranges.

Vitamin E: An antioxidant vitamin that was, until recently, commonly given to people with Alzheimer's. Most physicians discontinued prescribing vitamin E after a study linked it to an increased risk of dying.

BIBLIOGRAPHY

ARTICLES

AD2000 Collaborative Group, Long-term donepezil treatment in 565 patients with Alzheimer's disease (AD2000): randomized double-blind trial, *Lancet*, 2004; 363: 2105-15.

Alexopoulos, GS. et al. "Treatment of dementia and its behavioral disturbances." *A Postgraduate Medicine Special Report, from the Expert Consensus Guideline Series*, Jan. 2005, p. 101-108.

"Altered sense of smell could indicate Alzheimer's disease, new test." Dec. 14, 2004, online; http://www.medicalnewstoday.com.

"Alzheimer's disease vaccine a step nearer?" March 6, 2004, DrugResearcher.com, http://www.drugresearcher.com.

"Alzheimer's: when depression is a factor." Jan. 12, 2004, from MayoClinic.com, at http://www.cnn.com/Health/library.

"Alzheimer's researchers begin unique study of tangles," University Memory and Aging Center focuses on epilepsy drug." Press release by University Hospitals of Cleveland, Jan. 20, 2004, online; http://www.uhhs.com.

Ancoli-Israel, S. "Sleep and Alzheimer's disease." Undated, online; http://www.sleepfoundation.org.

Arnst, C. Alzheimer's: "Old Drug, New Hope." *BusinessWeek*, Feb. 3, 2005, online; www.businessweek.com.

Beeson, R. et al. "Loneliness and depression in caregivers of persons with Alzheimer's disease or related disorders." *Issues in Mental Health Nursing*, Dec. 2000, vol. 21, no. 8, p. 779-806.

Bird, T. "Genetic Factors in Alzheimer's Disease (editorial)." *New England Journal of Medicine*, March 3, 2005, vol. 352, no. 9, p. 862.

Butler S.M. et al. Age, "Education and changes in the Mini-Mental State Exam scores of older women: findings from the Nun Study." *Journal of the American Geriatrics Society*, June 1996, vol. 44, no. 6, p. 675-681.

"Choosing a specialty." American Medical Association, Dec. 6, 2004, online; http://www.ama-assn.org.

Cummings, J.L. "Treatment of Alzheimer's disease: current and future therapeutic approaches." *Review in Neurological Diseases*, vol. 1, no. 2, p. 60-69.

Davis, L.L. et al. "Biopsychological markers of distress in informal caregivers." *Biological Research for Nursing*. Oct. 2004, vol. 6, no. 2, p. 90-99.

Dimitra G. Georganopoulou DG et al. "Nanoparticle-based detection in cerebral spinal fluid of a soluble pathogenic biomarker for Alzheimer's disease." *Proceedings of the National Academy of Sciences*, Feb. 15, 2005, vol. 102, no. 7, p. 2273-2276.

Eastman, P. "Keeping Alzheimer's at bay: early diagnosis keeps patients functioning longer." March 2002, AARP Bulletin Online; http://www.aarp.org.

"Enhanced counseling, support interventions slashes long-term risk of depression among AD caregivers." Press release by the National Institutes of Health, May 1, 2004.

Fackelmann, K. "Minds in motion stay sharp." *USA Today*, Jan. 24, 2005.

"FDA approves memantine (Namenda) for Alzheimer's disease." Press release by the U.S. Food and Drug Administration, Oct. 17, 2003.

Geldmacher D.S., et al. "Donepezil is associated with delayed nursing home placement in patients with Alzheimer's disease." *Journal of the American Geriatric Society.* July 2003; vol. 51, no. 7, p. 937-44.

Gustafson, D. et al. "An 18-year follow-up of overweight and risk of Alzheimer disease." *Archives of Internal Medicine*, July 14, 2003, vol. 163, no. 13, p. 1524-1528.

"Health authorities reviewing safety data from investigational study involving reminyl (galantamine hydrobromide)." Press release, Jan. 21, 2005, online; http://www.us.reminyl.com.

"High homocysteine levels may double risk of dementia, Alzheimer's disease, new report suggests," Press release by the National Institute on Aging, Feb. 13, 2002.

Ingram, V. "Alzheimer's Disease: the molecular origins of the disease are coming to light, suggesting several novel therapies." *American Scientist*, July-August 2003, vol. 91. p. 312-321.

Kaufer, D.I. "Dementia with Lewy Bodies: Not exactly Alzheimer's or Parkinson's Disease." Summer 1997, Dear Friends newsletter, Alzheimer Disease Research Center at the University of Pittsburgh, reprinted online at www.alzheimers.org/pubs/dlb.htm.

Jensen M. et al. "Lifelong immunization human beta-amyloid (1-42) protects Alzheimer's transgenic mice against cognitive impairment throughout aging." *Neuroscience*, Nov. 23, 2004, vol. 130, no. 3, p. 667-684.

Leutwyler, K. "Toward early diagnosis of Alzheimer's disease." Scientific American.com, Aug. 13, 2001; http://sciam.com.

Lim, G. et al. "A Diet Enriched with the Omega-3 Fatty Acid Docosahexaenoic Acid Reduces Amyloid Burden in an Aged Alzheimer Mouse Model." *Journal of Neuroscience*, March 23, 2005, vol. 25, no. 12, p. 3032-3040.

Luchsinger J.A. et al. "Caloric intake and the risk of Alzheimer disease." *Archives of Neurology*, Aug. 2002, vol. 59, no. 8, p. 1258-63.

Lyketsos C.G. et al. "Treating depression in Alzheimer disease: efficacy and safety of sertraline therapy, and the benefits of depression reduction: the DIADS." *Archives of General Psychiatry*. July 2003, vol. 60, no. 7, p. 737-746.

"Memory and aging: Is losing my memory a normal part of aging?" Article at the University of Michigan Health System Web site, undated. online; http://www.med.umich.edu.

Mills, P.J. et al. "Vulnerable caregivers of Alzheimer disease patients have a deficit in beta2-adrenergic receptor sensitivity and density." *American Journal of Geriatric Psychiatry*, June 2004, vol. 12, no., p. 281-286.

Modrego P.J. et al. "Depression in patients with mild cognitive impairment increases the risk of developing dementia of Alzheimer type: a prospective cohort study." *Archives of Neurology*, August 2004, vol. 61, no. 8, p. 1290-1293.

Morris, M.C. et al. "Dietary Fats and the Risk of Incident Alzheimer Disease." *Archives of Neurology*, Feb. 2003, vol. 60, no. 2, p. 194-200.

"Nanoparticle technique detects Alzheimer's-related proteins." nanotechweb.org, Feb. 1, 2005; http://nanotechweb.org.

"Nanoscale diagnostic sets sights on Alzheimer's." Press release by National Science Foundation, Jan. 31, 2005, online; http://www.nsf.gov.

"National Institute on Aging, industry launch partnership, $60 million Alzheimer's disease neuroimaging initiative." Press release by the National Institutes of Health, Oct. 13, 2004.

Peterson, A. "A new approach to fighting Alzheimer's." *The Wall Street Journal*, June 29, 2004.

"Pittsburgh at the forefront of Alzheimer's research." University of Pittsburgh Medical Center. Press release, undated, online; http://healthjournal.upmc.com/0105/AlzheimerRsch.htm.

Rabheru, K. "Depression in dementia: diagnosis and treatment," *Psychiatric Times*, Nov. 2004, vol. 23, no. 13, online; http://www.psychiatrictimes.com.

Ramin, C.J. In search of lost time, *The New York Times Magazine*, Dec. 5, 2004.

Refolo L.M. et al. "Hypercholesterolemia accelerates the Alzheimer's amyloid pathology of transgenic mouse model." *Neurobiology of Disease*, Aug. 7, 2000 vol. 4, p. 321-331.

Reinberg, S. "Weight loss signals impending Alzheimer's," *Health-DayNews*. Jan. 10, 2005, online; http://health.yahoo.com/news.

"Researchers find definitive proof that repetitive head injury accelerate the pace of Alzheimer's." Press release, Jan. 15, 2002, University of Pennsylvania, online; http://www.upenn.edu.

"Saegis Pharmaceuticals begins phase II clinical trial of SGS742 for Alzheimer's disease." Press release, May 3, 2004, online; http://www.saegispharma.com.

"Safety concerns over galantamine; fallout from rofecoxib debacle grows." Alzheimer's Research Forum, Jan. 26, 2005, online; http://www.alzforum.org.

Scanlan J.M. et al. "Lymphocyte proliferation is associated with gender, caregiving, and psychosocial variables in older adults." *Journal of Behavioral Medicine*, Dec. 2001; vol. 24, no. 6, p. 537-559.

Schulz, R. et al. "Caregiving as a Risk Factor for Mortality, The Caregiver Health Effects Study." *Journal of the American Medical Association*, Dec.15, 1999, vol. 282, no. 23, p. 2215-2219.

Stewart, R. et al. "A 32-year prospective study of change in body weight and incident dementia; the Honolulu-Asia aging study." *Archives of Neurology*, Jan. 2005, vol. 62 no. 1, p. 55-60.

Teri, L. et. al. "Exercise plus behavioral management in patients with Alzheimer disease: a randomized controlled trial." *Journal of the American Medical Association*, Oct. 15, 2003; vol. 290, no. 15, p. 2015-2022.

"Trial of new type of drug that attacks amyloid." *Pharmaceutical News*, Nov. 4, 2004. online; http://www.news-medical.net/print_article.asp?id=6104.

VanGelder, B.M. et al. "Physical activity in relation to cognitive decline in elderly men; The FINE Study." *Neurology*, Dec. 28, 2004, vol. 63, no. 12, p.2316-2321.

Vitaliano, P.P. et al. "Is caregiving hazardous to one's physical health? A meta-analysis." *Psychological Bulletin*, 2003, vol. 129, no. 6, p. 946-972.

VonKanel R. et al. "Association of negative life event stress with coagulation activity in elderly Alzheimer caregivers." *Psychosomatic Medicine*, Jan.-Feb. 2003; vol. 65, no. 1, p. 145-150.

Whitmer R.A. et al. "Midlife cardiovascular risk factors and risk of dementia in late life." *Neurology*, Jan. 25, 2005. vol. 64, no. 2, p. 277-281.

Wisniewski K.E. et al. "Occurrence of neuropathological changes and dementia of Alzheimer's disease in Down's syndrome." *Annals of Neurology*, March 1985, vol. 17, no. 3, p. 278-282.

Yang, F. et al. "Curcumin inhibits formation of amyloid beta oligomers and fibrils, binds plaques, and reduces amyloid in vivo." *Journal of Biological Chemistry*, Feb. 18, 2005, vol. 280, no. 7, p. 5892-5901.

BOOKS

Castleman, Michael, Gallagher-Thompson, Dolores and Naythons, Matthew. *There's Still a Person in There: The Complete Guide to Treating and Coping With Alzheimer's.* New York, NY: Putnam Publishing Group, 2000.

Duyff, RL. *The American Dietetic Association's Complete Food and Nutrition Guide, 2nd edition.* Hoboken, NJ: Wiley & Sons, 2002.

Kuhn, Daniel. *Alzheimer's Early Stages: First Steps for Family, Friends and Caregivers.* Alameda, Calif.: Hunter House, 2003.

Mace, Nancy L., M.A. and Rabins, Peter V., M.D., MPh. *The 36-Hour Day: A Family Guide to Caring for Persons with Alzheimer's Disease, Related Dementing Illnesses and Memory Loss in Later Life.* Baltimore, MD: Johns Hopkins University Press, 1999.

Mittelman, Mary S., Dr., Ph., and Epstein, Cynthia, ACSW. *The Alzheimer's Healthcare Handbook.* New York: Marlowe & Co., 2002.

Petersen, Ronald, MD., PhD. ed, *Mayo Clinic on Alzheimer's Disease.* Rochester, Minn.: Mayo Clinic Health Information, 2002.

Shenk, David. *The Forgetting: Alzheimer's, Portrait of an Epidemic.* New York, NY: Anchor Books, 2003.

Shankle, William Rodman, M.S., M.D. and Amen, Daniel, M.D. *Preventing Alzheimer's: Ways to Help Prevent, Delay, Detect, and Even Halt Alzheimer's Disease and Other Forms of Memory Loss.* New York, NY: GP Putnam's, 2004. Reading, MA: Addison-Wesley Publishing Co., 1993.

GOVERNMENT PUBLICATIONS

"Alzheimer's Disease: Unraveling the mystery." December 2003; a publication by the National Institute on Aging.

"Choosing a Doctor." An online brochure of the National Institute on Aging, http://www.niapublications.org.

"2003 Progress Report on Alzheimer's Disease: Research advances at the NIH." October 2004; a publication by the National Institutes of Health and the National Institute on Aging.

WEB SITES

Alzheimer's Association: http://www.alz.org

Alzheimer's Disease Education and Referral Center: http://www.alzheimers.org

Alzheimer's Online (by Forest Pharmaceuticals, Inc.): http://www.alzheimersonline.com

The Alzheimer's Information Site: http://www.alzinfo.org

The Alzheimer Society of Canada: http://www.alzheimer.ca

Alzheimer's Foundation of America: http://www.alzfdn.org

American Academy of Family Physicians: http://www.familydoctor.org

American Geriatrics Society: http://www.americangeriatrics.org

American Neurological Association: http://aneuroa.org

American Psychiatric Association: http://www.psych.org

Anxiety Disorders Association of America: http://www.adaa.org

The Arc of the United States: http://www.thearc.org

Creuzfeldt-Jacob Disease Foundation Inc.: http://www.cjdfoundation.org

Elder Care Online: http://www.ec-online.net

eMedicine Consumer Health: http://www.emedicine.net

Family Caregiver Alliance: http://www.caregiver.org

Huntington's Disease Society of America: http://www.hdsa.org

MedicineNet.com: http://www.medicinenet.com

National Institute of Neurological Disorders and Stroke:
http://www.ninds.nih.gov

National Library of Medicine: http://medlineplus.gov/

Neurochem, Inc.: http://www.neurochem.com

Praecis Pharmaceuticals: http://www.praecis.com

Voyager Pharmaceuticals: http://www.voyagerpharm.com

webMD: http://www.webmd.com

Whonamedit.com: http://www.whonamedit.com

INDEX

ACKNOWLEDGMENTS

I would like to thank my editors Donna Raskin and Holly Schmidt for inviting me to write about a topic as intriguing and timely as Alzheimer's disease. I'd also like to thank the staff at Fair Winds for all their support, among them Ed Meagher and John Gettings.

I am grateful, too, to my collaborator Dr. Todd E. Feinberg for lending his medical expertise to this important project; and to Cliff Meirowitz for his help on the chapter on future planning.

In addition, I'd like to say thank you to Angela Yu, Nancy Cummings, Liz Pohlmann, and Diane VanDusen for giving me a close-up glimpse of Alzheimer's at the Marjorie Doyle Rockwell Center in Cohoes, N.Y. They took the time to open up their doors to me and gave me access to their wonderful library.

Special thanks need to go out to Chip and Sharon Gerber; Judy and Buddy Broadwater; Jeanne L. Lee; and Mary Lockhart, brave souls who came forward to share their stories about their experiences with Alzheimer's. Their stories taught me as much about the disease as any medical journal article did.

Finally, I must thank my family—Jeff, Samantha, and Annie—for simply being there.

—W.Y.

I wish to express my appreciation to the Gerald J. and Dorothy R. Friedman New York Foundation for Medical Research and its President Ms. Jane Friedman for their generous support of our research and clinical programs, and Betty and Morton Yarmon for their continuing support and guidance of our center.

—T.E.F.

ABOUT THE AUTHORS

Winnie Yu is a freelance writer and co-author of *What to Do When the Doctor Says It's Diabetes* and *What to Do When the Doctor Says It's Rheumatoid Arthritis*. Her work has appeared in numerous national publications including *Woman's Day, Reader's Digest, The Wall Street Journal,* and *Weight Watchers*. She has also contributed to several health books and written for the Web sites www.drugdigest.org and www.onemedicine.com.

Todd E. Feinberg, M.D., is Professor of Clinical Psychiatry and Neurology at Albert Einstein College of Medicine and Director of the Yarmon Neurobehavior and Alzheimer's Disease Center at Beth Israel Medical Center, in New York City. He is co-editor of *Behavioral Neurology and Neuropsychology* (McGraw-Hill), and has contributed to more than eighty articles, abstracts, or books. His most recent books are *Altered Egos: How the Brain Creates the Self* (Oxford) and the forthcoming *The Lost Self: Pathologies of the Brain and Identity* (with J. Keenan, Oxford, in press).

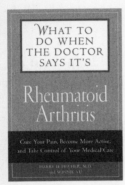

**WHAT TO DO WHEN
THE DOCTOR SAYS
IT'S RHEUMATOID ARTHRITIS**
By Harry D. Fishcer, M.D., and Winnie Yu
ISBN: 1-59233-146-7
$16.95/£10.99/$23.95 CAN
Paperback; 288 pages
Available wherever books are sold.

FINALLY, ANSWERS TO ALL YOUR QUESTIONS ABOUT RHEUMATOID ARTHRITIS!

Thanks to new medications and treatments, support groups, and self-management programs, millions of people diagnosed with rheumatoid arthritis (RA) have become more proactive in their own care. And early and aggressive treatment of RA has made it possible for many people to lead long, happy, and productive lives despite their diagnosis. Learning as much as possible about RA will give you greater confidence and control over your condition. Studies have shown that RA patients who are well-informed and actively participate in their own care have less pain and make fewer visits to the doctor than others with RA.

You'll learn:
• How to determine whether your health-care team is a good match for you
• Easy ways to keep track of your medical information so it's always handy
• Advice on sharing your diagnosis with your employer
• Travel and vacation tips that will ensure your time away is stress-free
• How to locate resources that offer the support you or your caregiver needs

About the Authors
Harry D. Fischer, M.D., is chief of the Division of Rheumatology at Beth Israel Medical Center and St. Luke's-Roosevelt Hospital Center, both in New York. He is also associate professor of clinical medicine at Albert Einstein College of Medicine.

Winnie Yu is a freelance writer who writes frequently about health and is coauthor of *What to Do When the Doctor Says It's Diabetes*

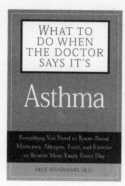

WHAT TO DO WHEN
THE DOCTOR SAYS IT'S ASTHMA
By Paul Hannaway, M.D.
ISBN: 1-59233-104-1
$16.95/£10.99/$23.95 CAN
Paperback; 288 pages
Available wherever books are sold.

A LEADING EXPERT SOLVES YOUR MOST COMMON BREATHING AND LIFESTYLE ISSUES.

Asthma affects hundreds of millions of people throughout the world and every day more of us are being diagnosed with this chronic, potentially debilitating illness. But with increased knowledge and new medical information, asthma patients can learn how to ease their symptoms and live worry-free, active lives. It is important to consider the particular air quality of the towns they live in, what types of medications and inhalers will work best for them, how to exercise to improve their health, and how to react to emergency breathing situations.

In *What To Do When The Doctor Says It's Asthma* you will learn more about:
• How to assemble a health-care team that is on your side and will help you achieve the medical results you want
• The latest research on asthma and new ways to reduce symptoms
• Alternative treatments that can diminish the occurrence of attacks
• How to help children with asthma

About the Author
Paul Hannaway, M.D., is an asthma suffer and father of two asthmatic children. He has treated thousands of patients with asthma and has authored numerous publications, including the American Medical Writers Award-winning *The Asthma Self-Help Book*.

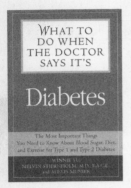

WHAT TO DO WHEN THE DOCTOR SAYS IT'S DIABETES
By Melvin Stjernholm, M.D., F.A.C.E.,
Winnie Yu, and Alexis Munier
$16.95/£10.99/$23.95 CAN
Paperback; 288 pages
Available wherever books are sold.

ARE YOU ONE OF THE TENS OF MILLIONS OF PEOPLE WHO HAVE BEEN DIAGNOSED WITH DIABETES?

In *What To Do When The Doctor Says It's Diabetes*, Dr. Melvin Stjernholm explains how to best care for yourself no matter what type of diabetes you are susceptible to, or currently have. Diabetes patients have many questions about medication, exercise, and especially diet
• Is it healthier to eat low-carb?
• Does everyone have to take insulin?
• Can exercise be dangerous if your blood-sugar levels are unreliable?
• How can I take care of myself so that I don't develop Type 2 diabetes?

This book answers all of these questions, and explains ways to improve your health based on the latest scientific findings.

About the Authors
Dr. Melvin Stjernholm, M.D., F.A.C.E. is an endocrinologist who has been in private practice in Boulder, Colorado for the past thirty years. He is board certified in endocrinology, diabetes, and metabolism, and holds an appointment as Clinical Professor of Medicine at the University of Colorado.

Winnie Yu is a freelance writer focusing on health and parenting for national publications including *Woman's Day*, *Weight Watchers*, and *Parents*, as well as the Web site drugdigest.org. Her work has also appeared in *Reader's Digest* and *The Wall Street Journal*, and she has contributed to several health books published by Rodale Inc.

Alex Munier is a writer and opera singer diagnosed with diabetes at age 13.